WOMEN'S HEALTH

Also by Penny Kane

ASKING DEMOGRAPHIC QUESTIONS (*editor with David Lucas*)
CHINA'S ONE-CHILD FAMILY POLICY (*editor with Delia Davin
    and Elisabeth Croll*)
THE CHOICE GUIDE TO BIRTH CONTROL (*with John Porter*)
CHOICE NOT CHANCE: A Handbook of Fertility Control
    (*with Beula Bewley and Judith Cook*)
CONSUMER GUIDE TO BIRTH CONTROL
    (*with Margaret Sparrow*)
DIFFERENTIAL MORTALITY: Methodological Issues and
    Biosocial Factors (*edited with Lado Ruzicka and
    Guillaume Wunsch*)
EHKAISY [Contraception]
FAMINE IN CHINA 1959–61: Demographic and
    Social Implications
THE SECOND BILLION: People and Population in China
SUCCESSFULLY EVER AFTER (*with Shirley Sloan Fader*)
TRADITION, DEVELOPMENT AND THE INDIVIDUAL
    (*edited with Lado T. Ruzicka*)
THE WHICH? GUIDE TO BIRTH CONTROL

Women's Health

From Womb to Tomb

Penny Kane

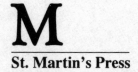

St. Martin's Press

First edition 1991
Reprinted 1992
Second edition 1994

Published in Great Britain by
THE MACMILLAN PRESS LTD
Houndmills, Basingstoke, Hampshire RG21 2XS
and London
Companies and representatives
throughout the world

A catalogue record for this book is available
from the British Library.

ISBN 0–333–52287–7 hardcover
ISBN 0–333–61517–4 paperback

Printed in Great Britain by
Mackays of Chatham PLC
Chatham, Kent

First published in the United States of America 1991 by
Scholarly and Reference Division,
ST. MARTIN'S PRESS, INC.,
175 Fifth Avenue,
New York, N.Y. 10010

ISBN 0–312–04635–9 (cloth)
ISBN 0–312–10623–8 (paper)

Library of Congress Cataloging-in-Publication Data
Kane, Penny.
Women's health from womb to tomb / Penny Kane
p. cm.
Includes bibliographical references and index.
ISBN 0–312–04635–9 (cloth) — ISBN 0–312–10623–8 (paper)
1. Women—Health and hygiene. I. Title.
RA564.85.K36 1991
613'.0424—dc20   90–32946
                                            CIP

Contents

List of Tables

List of Figures

Acknowledgements

It would have been impossible to write this book without two sources of information, above all. The first is the World Health Organisation, which not only collects a vast amount of material on the health of the different countries of the world, but which analyses much of it to identify major trends, problems, developments and puzzles. The publications of WHO have been invaluable, but I am also grateful for the personal support of Dr Alan Lopez, of the Global Epidemiological Surveillance and Health Situation Assessment Division.

The other major source of material is the Office of Population, Censuses and Surveys, in Britain. Britain has one of the best – if not the best – systems of demographic and health data in the world. It is not just that OPCS collects a great deal of information, but that it publishes it (generally) promptly and in very useable forms. And HMSO are equally prompt in fulfilling orders to the other side of the world. I am also grateful to Virginia Blakey, then of the University College Cardiff Population Centre for sifting through much OPCS material for earlier years for me.

The continuing care of Bruce Hunter and his colleagues at David Higham Associates both initiated the book and kept me working at it.

My greatest source of help and support has been my husband, Lado Ruzicka. He encouraged me to write the book and taught me most of what I know about epidemiology and demography. He is not, of course, responsible for the bits I don't know or for any inaccuracies or misinterpretations.

Introduction

The idea for this book came from an initial suggestion that I might like to write a book on some aspect of 'women's health'. Books on women's health have focused, effectively, on the health of women during the reproductive years, or on some aspect of health which is specific to women – the menopause, or childbearing, for instance. A large number of books have been produced, by people varying as much in their approaches as do Derek Llewellyn-Jones and the Boston Women's Cooperative; among them virtually everybody can find something which they will enjoy and which will satisfy their demand for information and/or reassurance.

As I thought about the subject, though, I began to feel that the reproductive focus was rather a narrow definition of women's health, and one which left out many of the great differences between men and women from the time of conception to death.

Of course, the question of defining health at all is an extremely difficult one. The World Health Organisation describes health as 'a state of complete mental, physical and social wellbeing, and not merely the absence of disease or infirmity'. Which is a nice ideal, but impossible to measure. So all studies of health have to operate by trying to quantify its opposite: ill-health, disease, disability and death. The amount of ill-health can be assessed from statistics – on visits to a general practitioner or specialist, hospitalisation, or causes of death, for example – or from surveys. From these manifestations of ill-health or health impairments we draw conclusions about the health status or health situation of a group, rather than of individuals: women and men of a given age; occupation; education; marital status; and so on. But whether there is a direct connection between declines in deaths, or in visits to a GP, and improvements in real health is a debatable point. Reductions in death rates may mean the survival of some people whose functional health is impaired. Such reductions defer the inevitable – death – to an older age. Whether the years added to life are full of complete mental, physical and social well-being is another question.

In the absence of a better measure, however, there are two ways in which you can look at the health of women. One is to examine their *health situation* by collecting up information on the types of illness they get, the ages at which they are likely to die, and so on. That will give you a straightforward picture of women's health and of health risks.

More girls than boys are born, in the first place, and some congenital diseases are more common to – or only occur in – one or the other sex. In their teens and early twenties, women have less illness and death from accidents and violence than men, but suffer more from things like anorexia, as well as having problems with menstruation and pregnancy. Adult women have a different pattern of accidents to men, and often different industrial injuries; they also have different patterns of mental illness. All these are in addition to their childbearing, contraceptive and reproductive problems. And as they get older, women die from a slightly different group of diseases to men: their cancers, for instance, are not the same. Finally, and most importantly, women also live longer, and are more likely to spend their last years alone with the disabilities of old age.

The other way of approaching women's health is to look at the *health status* of women. Status can only be measured by comparison with the status of another group, and the obvious group is men. By comparing particular aspects of women's health situation with that of men, you can see which sex has greater risk of particular types of illness or handicap, or at which ages those risks are greater. From those statistics, you can also compare the different health situation of different groups of women – women of different social classes, for example, or women in different countries.

Either type of comparison may be, on its own, insufficient or misleading. There are certain diseases or causes of deaths which men don't get and women do – no man dies of childbearing, for instance – and others which men risk and women don't. So where there are biological differences, a comparison between the sexes is not really comparing like with like. On the other hand, unless you compare one group of women with another group of women, you cannot be sure that the differences are really biological, rather than the result of particular social or economic or cultural circumstances. If you look at many developing countries, you will see that women in their reproductive years have a higher death rate than men, because of the extra risk of death that childbearing produces. But if you look at the richer countries of the world, you will find that the extra risk of death to women in those reproductive years has almost disappeared. So the risk of death is not purely a biological one; it is a combination of the fact that women have babies and of the fact that in some societies they have them in conditions which add very considerably to their vulnerability.

This is a fairly obvious example. There is, however, a wide variety of occasions where it is impossible to tell whether, or how far, a health difference between the sexes is based on biology: English men over age 65 have higher rates of death from ischaemic heart disease than women in the same age group, but although it is thought that lifestyle (amount of exercise, smoking, drinking and so on) plays part in this difference, we don't yet know whether it is responsible for all of the difference, or whether there are underlying biological or other mechanisms which play a part as well.

Neither is it easy to define those social and economic conditions which play a part in health differences between different groups of women, or women and men. It is usually easier to show that women in a lower social class have a worse health status than women in a higher one, or women in the third world a worse one than women in Europe, than it is to explain why that should be or how the difference can be eliminated. For one thing, social and economic conditions are usually not single states but a jumble of circumstances. A poor woman will quite often be an uneducated one; she is more likely to live in inadequate housing and in a more polluted environment; she is less likely to have an adequate diet; and so on. Whether there is one particular circumstance in all of these which is the overriding threat to her health it is often impossible to discover. Often the suspicion is that the risk results from a combination of things – that her poor education means she is less hygiene-conscious and less knowledge-able about diet; that poor nutrition means she is more susceptible to infections; that those infections are more common in a crowded and poor environment; that her lack of education and status make her less likely to seek early treatment.

I thought it would be interesting, in the first place, to see exactly what women's health status consisted of, and how it might be changing. Without that kind of overall picture of how women live, or die, and exactly how they are advantaged or disadvantaged, either by comparison with other groups of women or with men, how can we know what we should be fighting to improve? Our feminist priorities have traditionally concentrated on aspects of fertility and its control, because these were the first and most obvious manifestation of the special needs of women. In many parts of the world, they still represent a major problem: there are too many women who still die during their reproductive years and would love to survive long enough to chance dying of cancer. But, in Europe, in Australasia, or North America, the major health problems of women today may be very different, as I hope I have shown in this book.

Secondly – and this is linked with how one solves those health problems – I wanted to find out *why* women's health was so different from men's, in so many ways. This turned out to be a much more difficult question to come to grips with: the answer, in most cases, seems to be that nobody really knows. There are a few genetic influences which have been identified, and a suspicion of more to be found – assuming that legislation on things like research on very early embryos, for example, does not make more research impossible, which would be a pity as the genetic conditions are among the most heartbreaking and difficult to deal with. There are some biological influences, though fewer than one might suppose. Many of the answers came down to 'behavioural' factors – a vague term covering everything from stress levels, to what you eat and drink, to what you wear. These behavioural influences are usually all mixed up so that it is extremely difficult to identify any particular one, or particular 'mix', as being responsible for any specific event. It is high time doctors and social scientists learnt to work together to understand the behavioural bases for differential health.

All this means that I have often raised more questions than I have answered, and the best one can say for that, I suppose, is that it may encourage somebody to try and find the answers.

I also wanted to write the book in such a way that it made sense to the non-specialist. Most of the material on which it is based comes from demographic, epidemiological or sociological texts which are fairly specialised even within their own fields. They also tend to discuss only a limited number of the aspects of different health between males and females. I hoped that by presenting that research in a more comprehensive framework, and in a way that can be understood, it would make the picture clearer to all those interested in women's health issues: policy makers and those working in community health and the general reader alike.

This book is divided into two parts. The first sections look at women's health in a general perspective, concentrating primarily on the countries of Europe but using developing world countries to show how similar they may be or what changes have taken place in our Western achievement of a greater length of life. Chapter 1 sets the scene by describing the overall patterns of women's health by comparison with those of men – how long they live, at which particular ages they have the greatest health advantage or disadvantage, and how these trends have changed or are changing over time. It provides the basic demographic background and explains some of the basic concepts which are used in the book. Chapter 2 looks at some of the theories which have been put forward to explain women's generally better longevity. Illness, rather than death, is the focus of the third chapter: how the amount and types of illness vary between men and women and some of the explanations as to why women should have generally higher rates. It also looks at the differential use of health services by men and women. Chapter 4 primarily compares women with women – examining how far these overall trends in women's health are universally valid for women and how far they arise from social and economic characteristics.

The second part of the book concentrates in much more detail on examining differences between women and men at different ages or stages of life. I have used largely British material in these remaining chapters, for several reasons. There is a great deal of information available for Britain, and it is generally processed quite quickly, so that the statistics reflect current events. What is more, the health statistics broadly cover the population, which is less often the case elsewhere. The existence of a National Health Service makes this possible. In countries where there are a large number of private doctors and hospitals, comprehensive data are more difficult to collect and less likely to be available. Obviously, figures for Britain (or England and Wales, or England alone) cannot be extrapolated exactly to other European or industrialised countries: there are variations by region even within England, for that matter. All the same, while women in some countries may have rather higher or lower rates of illness or death from one particular cause than they do in England, the broad pattern of women's health is unlikely to be radically different. The early chapters show, in fact, just how much overall similarity countries with a high life expectation have.

In these later chapters the major causes of death (and where possible disease) are described for each stage of life for both sexes: this gives us the overall epidemiology. Where those causes of death differ for the two sexes, the difference is identified and reasons suggested. I should stress that this is not a directory of all the possible conditions which may affect men and women; neither is it a do-it-yourself health guide. I have concentrated only on identifying those things which are likely to affect most of us, one way and another: the main patterns of illness and of death at different ages. I believe it is only in that kind of a context that we can see what women's health through life consists of, and judge the relative risks to it. Without that framework, it is difficult to evaluate the benefits and costs of different interventions, from contraception to diet, and impossible to plan really effective ways of ensuring we get the most out of our lives.

Looking at the detailed picture of men's and women's health at different ages in Britain also helps to answer some of the questions which were raised in earlier chapters, especially in Chapter 3. Women have long been believed to suffer – or to complain of – worse health than men, despite their longer expectation of life. This phenomenon has been used to explain those longer lives, with the suggestion that women are more health-conscious and take action earlier than men to prevent or limit conditions which would otherwise lead to death. Alternatively, it has been used to suggest that women fuss more about their health when it is really perfectly good as their life expectation shows. A third explanation has been that women really do have more illness than men but are nevertheless somehow more enduring and manage to survive it.

The analysis in Chapters 5–7 suggests that the truth is both simpler, and more complicated, than any of the existing theories. The extra use women make of hospitals and doctors, and the greater ill-health they report, is largely restricted to particular age-groups. Much of the apparent over-representation of women in the statistics results from women's unique obstetric and gynaecological needs, and when these are taken into account, their general health profile differs much less sharply from that of men. Some of the remaining excess comes from the different risks men and women face at different ages. What remains – and it is a comparatively small proportion – is largely concentrated in a few areas, where the diagnoses are unfortunately ambiguous. Taken together, they may imply some unrecognised stress-related problems of women's health, and a need for much more careful studies of these.

Introduction to the Second Edition

Women's health, as a topic for discussion, research and policy initiatives, seems to have become much more prominent in the two years since
Women's Health: From Womb to Tomb was first published. Naturally I
am all in favour of this development, at least in principle; if I had not
thought women's health deserved more attention than it was getting, I
should not have bothered to write the book. All the same, I am not as
happy as I might be about some of the ways in which the subject is being
approached.

First of all, I still consider that 'women's health' is being interpreted
in a very narrow sense. The term itself remains largely synonymous with
'women's reproductive health' as though there are no particular health
issues, or health differences, outside those which are related to women's
childbearing function. In this narrow interpretation, the term also
suggests that concerns about women's health are limited to the years
between puberty and the menopause. Such an approach ignores the very
real distinctions between males and females in the patterns of illness,
accidents and causes of deaths. It ignores, too, the fact that these
differences exist at all times: in childhood, in maturity and in old age.

In addition, much of the discussion about women's health, as well as
the research being undertaken to improve our understanding of what that
involves, seems to be confined to a rather limited range of issues.
Analysis of the research being carried out in Australia, for example,*
suggests that even the umbrella term 'reproductive health' is misleadingly comprehensive. Most of the work going on under that heading
focuses upon pregnancy, childbirth, fertility (especially contraception)
and infertility. Other widely experienced health problems related to
women's reproductive system – menstrual pain, for instance, or cystitis
– remain ignored. Research involving the health of older women (and
there was not a lot of it in progress) had only two specific themes:
osteoporosis and urinary incontinence. The rapid growth of interest in
hormone replacement therapy has – since that analysis of research
projects was completed – probably added a third theme.

Even so, there is surely more to the health of older women than these research efforts would suggest.

The vast majority of the research projects investigating women's health – and an even greater proportion of the money involved – concentrates on biomedical research. To some extent that is inevitable; biomedical research is certainly needed, and it is expensive. But many of those feminists working in the women's health field argue (and I would agree with them) that health is not just a question of specific medical conditions; it is significantly dependent on individuals' general well-being and confidence in their ability to control their world and their relationships within that world. As a result, there are increasing calls for studies that link women with their environmental setting.

Potentially, this could bring greater results in understanding of a whole range of women's health problems. I suspect that it could be particularly important in shedding light on some of the stresses which affect women particularly in middle and later life, and which are discussed in Chaper 7. But I do want to enter a small caveat. We need to be careful that studies of 'women in the family context', for instance, do not end up by concentrating on the needs or functions of the family group as a whole, at the expense of the individual women. Maternal and child policies and programmes provide a generally dismal example of what can happen. Too frequently, those programmes have only addressed the health of the mother when, and in so far as, it might affect the child's survival. The demands and concerns of the women have been subsumed by those of their children.

Finally, I should perhaps make it clear to potential readers that, while this book has a feminist perspective, it does not attempt a feminist theory of women's health. In writing a book like this, there are at least two possible approaches. One – which was mine – was to start from a fairly straightforward assumption that by looking in as much detail as possible at the statistical evidence about women's health at all ages, and in poorer as well as richer countries, it would be feasible to see how far it was different from the health profile of men, and how far any differences were intrinsic rather than socioeconomic or cultural. I was looking, in other words, for a distinct profile of women's health.

The alternative perspective is to start from a theory about the 'why' of any differences and then see how far the available evidence supports or contradicts it. That is possibly a more ambitious approach but it does depend on there being an explicit recognition that real differences exist in the first place. Except in reproductive health matters, such recognition of the separateness of women's health has not been widespread. I hope

that *Women's Health: From Womb to Tomb* contributes to our understanding of differences; I hope even more that it will encourage others
to debate the 'why' of those differences. It is those debates which may
bring closer the goal of women's health as a state of 'complete mental,
physical and social well-being'.

Penny Kane
Major's Creek, July 1993

*Kane, Penny (1991) *Researching Women's Health: An Issues Paper
for the Department of Health, Housing and Community Services*,
Australian Government Publishing Service, Canberra
  I use this Australian analysis as an example simply because it exists;
although the topics of research might be different elsewhere, I suspect
that the overall pattern of narrowly-focused research on a few limited
aspects of women's health would not be significantly different.

1 Trends in Women's Health

That there are differences in health between men and women has been noticed, and those differences studied, for more than 300 years. One of the earliest scholars to discuss the issue was an Englishman, John Graunt, in 1662. He analysed the weekly reports of deaths in the parishes of London, and reported that the proportional numbers of deaths of women were below those of men (Graunt, 1975).

> Yet I have heard *Physicians* say, that they have two women patients to one man, which Assertion seems very likely; for that women have either the *Greensickness*, or other like Distempers, are sick of *Breedings*, *Abortions*, *Child-bearing*, *Sorebreasts*, *Whites*, *Obstructions*, *Fits of the Mother* and the like.

The reason, he concluded, for their better survival record was either that the doctors managed to cure women of their many illnesses, or that '. . .men, being more intemperate than women, die as much by reason of their Vices, as women do by the Infirmitie of their *Sex*'.

A recent comment on Graunt's explanation is that 'it embodies most if not all of the principal elements underlying current theories of the sex mortality differential' (Lopez, 1984a).

But why, when writing a book about the health of women, begin with death? The answer is, in the first place, that deaths – their relative frequency and causes – are the best indicator we have of a community's health. There is much more material recorded about numbers of deaths and what people die from than there is about their illnesses. There are perfectly sensible reasons for this.

In the first place, the fact of death is striking and incontestable. We can all recognise that it has happened; we all accept its importance, because of its finality. Also, numbers of deaths are – at least in countries with a reasonable vital registration system – fairly easy to count.

1

Causes of death are rather more difficult. Does one register the immediate cause which may be, for example, pneumonia? Or does one recognise the underlying cause, which may, in the case of an elderly person, be a simple broken hip, or a more complicated history of emphysema and/or bronchitis? Does the diagnosis come from what the doctor believes, or from what a post-mortem actually shows?

The agreed procedures on defining causes of death, which are internationally accepted and used in reporting death, are that the doctor puts on the certificate both the disease or condition which *directly* leads to death, and any other antecedent causes or conditions which contributed to it. One of these will be the 'underlying cause of death' and that is the one which will be reported, and shown in the statistics on causes of death, if it is different from the immediate cause. Inevitably, some doctors are better at, or more careful about, filling in death certificates than others. Where coroners are involved, in some places they are appointed from the legal profession; in others they are doctors; which type of qualification they have may also affect their reporting. Overall, however, the statistics reflect the facts reasonably well.

Where death is concerned, it is much easier to get agreement about what the figures mean. In the case of illness, what does one measure? The number of hospital cases? Or family practitioner visits? Or surveys of people's own perceptions? We shall, indeed, be looking at all these, but it has to be admitted that they have their limitations as indications of what health is all about. Whereas death is, at least, the ultimate manifestation of illness or accident.

The first, and most important, way of measuring the health status of a community or of groups within a community is by looking at how long, on average, they are likely to live.

LIFE EXPECTATION AT BIRTH

Life expectation at birth is a measure which summarises the current frequency and age pattern of deaths in the form of a single index. It implies that a population born in the year of the measure can be expected – if conditions remain unchanged – to survive, on average, a particular number of years. It is often said to be the best single measure of a country's overall 'development', because the progress made in extending the expected length of life reflects not only economic conditions but levels of health, education, the status of women, and so on.

In a poor country, the better-off sections of the community in cities may have a life expectation which is more or less similar to that of people in the industrialised world – but the presence of vast numbers of peasants or slum-dwellers without access to enough food, health care, education and so on will be reflected in a national life expectation which is much lower. In that sense, average national life expectation is likely to give a similar picture of the socio-economic conditions of the country to an indicator like Gross National Product per head. Life expectation may be a more realistic indicator, though, because it does cover the whole of society, whereas GNP disregards many contributions to the economy such as women's unpaid work, in the home or elsewhere.

Although in this sense the measure of life expectation reflects what could be called 'quality of life' there is another sense in which it does not. In countries with an already high life expectation, pushing it up still further may mean prolonging the lives of the very old, but not necessarily prolonging their capacity to lead a reasonably healthy and independent existence. This is discussed in more detail in Chapter 3. The point to remember here is that there is currently a great debate about whether there is some 'natural' biological limit to length of life (say around 100 years for most people) or whether, with the right kinds of care, most of us could go on living for considerably longer periods. Bound up with this controversy is the linked question of what gains in life expectation really mean: are we adding years to life, or life to years? If the former, many people would question the benefits of further extending it.

Like any single national figure, national life expectation at birth is an average which hides considerable differences between individuals and different groups of the population. To understand what is happening within those groups, and whether some are missing out or others doing considerably better than might be expected, you have to look at the different life expectation that each group has. The most common ways of looking at these differences are by examining the life expectation by

> social class;
> geographical area (urban/rural, poorer
> districts versus richer, and so on);
> and by sex.

We shall begin by looking at life expectation by sex in some of the wealthier countries of the world, to see how women make out compared to men in countries where there is generally a long expectation of life.

WOMEN'S BETTER LIFE EXPECTATION IN EUROPE

Graunt's observation that women lived longer than men is broadly still true today. In most countries, though, women not only live longer, but are actually *increasing* the gap between their life expectation and that of men. That gap is now around 6.5 years in the industrialised countries of the world.

TABLE 1.1 *Trends in longevity: life expectation at birth in selected European countries around 1960, 1970 and 1980*

| | Life expectation at birth | | | | | |
| | males | | | females | | |
Country	1960	1970	1980	1960	1970	1980
Belgium	66.3	67.3	69.0	72.2	73.5	75.6
Czechoslovakia	67.8	66.2	67.5	73.2	72.9	74.6
England & Wales	68.2	69.1	70.2	74.2	75.4	76.2
Finland	65.4	66.7	68.9	72.6	75.2	77.2
German Dem. Republic	66.5	68.1	68.7	71.4	73.3	74.8
Greece	67.3	70.1	72.9	70.4	73.6	77.6
Hungary	66.4	66.8	66.0	70.6	72.6	73.2
Netherlands	71.1	71.2	72.4	75.9	77.2	78.9
Norway	71.0	71.4	72.3	76.0	77.7	78.7
Porgugal	61.6	64.6	67.3	67.3	71.0	74.2
Sweden	71.2	72.2	72.8	74.9	77.1	78.8

SOURCE: Lopez, 1984

Looking at the life expectations in Europe (Table 1.1), you can see a variety of patterns. The first, and most obvious, is that women, even at the beginning of the period covered by the table, did better than men. Only in Portugal did they, around 1960, have an expectation of life below 70 years. By contrast, in only three countries – the Netherlands, Norway and Sweden – did men have a life expectation above 70 years.

Twenty years later, men had reached a life expectation of more than 70 years in only two more countries (England and Wales, and Greece). By the same date, around 1980, women in most of the countries had a life expectation above 75 years.

It is also clear from the table that some of the biggest gains, for both sexes, have been in the poorer countries – Portugal and Greece. But even here women have done better than men: in Portugal they gained 6.9 years compared with 5.7 years for men, and in Greece they gained 7.6 years to the men's 5.6 years.

A third point about Table 1.1 is that women's life expectation has shown steady progress in every single country, while the same is not true for men. In Czechoslovakia and Hungary, conditions for males appear to have actually *deteriorated* since around 1960. In the Netherlands, Norway and Sweden, conditions for males have only improved slightly. It could be argued that the latter group of countries had such good life expectation at the beginning of the period that further improvement could hardly be assumed – but the trends for women in those same countries have not got stuck in the same way.

WOMEN'S LIFE EXPECTATION IN DEVELOPING COUNTRIES

The reasons for these differences between women's and men's life expectation are discussed later in this chapter. First, though, we can look at life expectation in some of the developing countries of the world, to see whether the pattern of overall female advantage in life expectation has a universal validity. A problem in doing this is that very few developing countries collect the kind of statistics needed for a reliable calculation. As a result, demographers have had to design 'models' for the different regions.

These models involve groupings of countries with similar mortality patterns – not all of them geographically within the region to which their mortality characteristics assign them – which are based on such data as are available, and assumptions from those data. The United Nations Population Division (1983) have produced a table which

an indication of the difference between female and male life expectation at birth for areas with a different overall life expectation.

TABLE 1.2   *Female minus male life expectation at birth (in years)*

Regions	Life expectation at birth (both sexes combined)			
	40 years	*50 years*	*60 years*	*70 years*
(Models of the United Nations)				
Latin America	2.3	3.3	4.0	4.6
South Asia	−2.9	−0.8	1.4	3.5
Far East Asia	–	–	6.8	7.1
(Models of Coale and Demeny)				
West Region	2.7	2.9	3.6	4.0
North Region	3.1	3.4	3.7	3.7
East Region	2.9	3.4	4.1	4.7
South Region	1.7	2.8	3.8	3.9

SOURCE: United Nations Population Division, 1983

This Table 1.2 shows two things, basically. The first is that when
you subtract male from female life expectation, you are almost
always left with a plus figure – in other words, that women show
additional years of life and that this is true in countries where the
average life expectation is very low (around 40 years) as well as where
it is high (around 70 years). Here too, as in Europe, *women are living
longer than men*.

There are differences between the regions in how many extra years
of life women have, at different levels of life expectation. But the
other thing the table shows is that, reading across the columns, in
every region the number of extra years of life women have compared
with men goes up at every level of life expectation. In other words, as
both sexes gain additional years, women tend to gain *more* additional
years.

One developing country for which there are good statistics is China
(Table 1.3), and it provides an interesting example of how rapidly

women make these extra gains when the health of a population begins to improve. Average life expectation at birth in China roughly doubled between 1949 and 1981 but that average masks quite considerable differences between richer and poorer provinces, and urban and rural areas, in this huge country of over 1000 million people.

TABLE 1.3   *Life expectation at birth in China, 1981, by rural/urban residence and sex*

	China	Cities	Towns	Rural
Total	67.60	70.63	71.30	66.89
Male	66.17	68.93	69.45	65.51
Female	69.06	72.42	73.28	68.27
Female advantage	2.89	3.49	3.83	2.76

SOURCE: Liu Zheng, 1986

While life expectation for men in towns exceeds that of men in the rural areas by almost four years, women in towns show an advantage in life expectation of five years. (The slightly higher expectation of life in towns than in large cities is presumably due to the lower level of pollution, motor accidents and so on.)

WOMEN'S LIFE EXPECTATION WORLDWIDE

So it seems fair to say that, looking at both developed and developing countries, *women live longer than men.*

The only region where this does not hold true is South Asia, because among the countries considered in the model were some from the Indian sub-continent, which have had lower female than male life expectation: India, Pakistan, Bangladesh, Burma, Nepal, probably Afghanistan, and, until the early 1960s, Sri Lanka. Why those countries should be exceptions to the general rule is something which we will be able to examine further on. Before that, we need to break down the overall figures for life expectation, to see what they imply at different stages of existence.

DEATH RATES AT DIFFERENT AGES

Life expectation at birth for a given year or period is, as we saw, a measure which implies that a population born in that year can expect to survive, on average, a particular number of years. We can now look at the *pattern of survival* behind this overall measure, and identify how that pattern is different for men and women.

In order to do this, we need the number of deaths for each 1000 people at different ages along the whole life span. Those measures are called *age-specific mortality rates*.

Both in countries with high, and those with low, life expectations the curve on a graph of age-specific mortality is U-or J-shaped. That is, it shows high mortality in the first year of life and in early childhood, and again at the older ages. In developing countries with very high infant and child mortality, the curve will be more of a 'U'; in the Western world, where most deaths have now been postponed to old age, it looks more like a 'J' (Figure 1.1).

WOMEN'S DEATH RATES AT DIFFERENT AGES

In addition to the different shapes of the curves depending on how large a proportion of deaths occur in childhood, curves for men and women also differ from each other. This indicates different health risks for each sex at different ages.

In the industrialised countries, men have higher death rates throughout their life span. There are two phases of the life cycle in which the differences are at their maximum. These are between the ages of 15 and 24, when male mortality is on average about 2.7 times the rate for women, and again after age 45, where death rates are typically double those for women. A common way of showing the different death rates is to measure the amount of *excess* mortality, for one sex compared to the other, by using a *ratio* of male to female mortality rates, age by age.

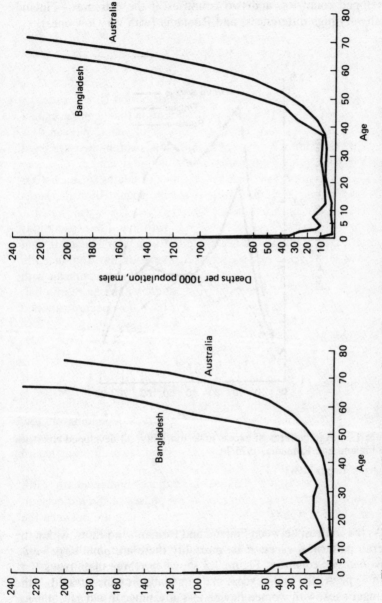

Figure 1.1 Age specific mortality rates for males and females, Australia 1981/2 and Bangladesh, 1983.

SOURCE: Australian Government Actuary, 1985, and Shaik et. al., 1985

Figure 1.2 shows the average age profile of excess male mortality in developed countries, and two countries at the extremes – Finland (with very high differences) and Romania (with very low ones).

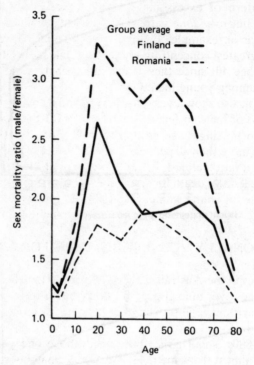

Figure 1.2   Age patterns of excess male mortality, all developed countries and Finland and Romania, 1975/78.

SOURCE: Lopez, 1983.

As the contrast between Finland and Romania indicates, within the overall pattern of excess male mortality there are quite large *variations between countries*. Figure 1.3 shows the three main types.

In Type A, the main excess male mortality is concentrated in the younger ages, with women having less advantage in old age; there is only one peak in the curve. Types B and C have similar double-

peaked curves, but in Type B the high peak at the younger ages is
much steeper than in Type C, so that in Switzerland, for example, the
deaths among young men are about 3.3 times as high as those for
young women, while in England and Wales there are only some 2.4
excess male deaths at the same ages.

The pattern of excess male mortality varies not just between
countries, but *over time* within any particular country. If you take
Australia as an example, Figure 1.4 shows that between 1881 and
1922, the greatest concentration of excess male mortality among men
was after age 40; since then it has increasingly switched to excess
mortality among young men.

The graph also shows, very clearly, what an increase there has been
in the ratio of male to female death rates over the past century. In
1881–90, in no single age group did male mortality exceed that of
females by more than 40 per cent (ratio 1.4); by 1980–82 no single age
group had a ratio *below* 1.7. In other words, at the beginning of the
period, the risks of death for young men were no more than two-fifths
above those for young women. By 1980–82, young men had a risk of
death more than three times the rate for women of the same age.

TRADITIONALLY VULNERABLE AGES FOR WOMEN

The changes in the Australian ratios of male to female death rates at
different ages over time give us the first clues as to why women in so
many countries have improved their life expectation more than have
men.

In the 1880s, small girls (those aged above one year to around
eight) had almost the same risks of death as small boys, as the graph
indicates: the ratio of their respective mortality rates was only just
above one. Since then, girls have gained rapidly. Until after World
War II, the ratios were close to one in the ages 20–35, which means
that declines in mortality were about the same for men and women in
those age-groups. After the 1940s, females in those age-groups began
to improve their position.

In other words, it seems that *traditionally, small girls and women in
the reproductive years may have had a greater vulnerability* than exists
today. Changes which have reduced the risks of death in those two
phases of women's lives may have been a major factor in giving
women a longer life expectation than men. Such specific changes, in
addition to the range of health benefits which affected both sexes

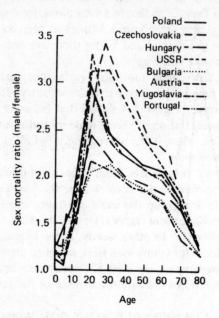

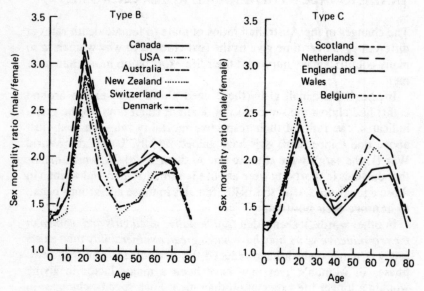

Figure 1.3   Age patterns of male excess mortality for various groups of developed countries, 1975/78.

SOURCE: Lopez, 1983.

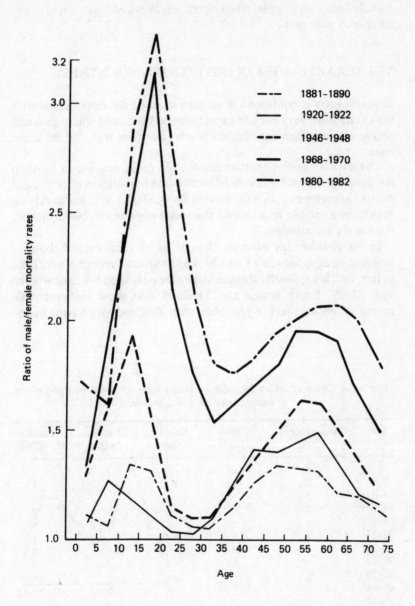

Figure 1.4　Sex ratios of mortality rates, by sex: Australia, selected periods 1980/90 and 1980/82.

SOURCE:　Australian Government Actuary, 1985.

equally, may also have given them an improved life expectation compared with men.

VULNERABLE AGES IN DEVELOPING COUNTRIES

This suspicion is confirmed if we turn to some developing countries which still have very low life expectation at birth, and where girls and young women often have higher death rates than males of the same ages.

The data for such countries are not always as reliable as those in the developed world, because of inadequate registration of births and deaths. Sometimes – as is the case in Bangladesh – one has to rely on data from a sample area, rather than total population. Nevertheless, the results are striking.

In Bangladesh, for example, female death rates exceed those of males at all ages between 1 and 39, and Pakistan's record is very little better. In China, death rates are higher for girls aged 1–4, and women ages 25–29. South Korea and Thailand also show higher female mortality among the 1–4 year olds, with Thailand also having excess

TABLE 1.4   *Ages at which life table mortality rates of females exceed those of males: selected Asian countries*

Age	Bangladesh 1982	China 1981	Korea 1980	Thailand 1973/4	Pakistan 1976/9
0	–	–	–	–	–
1–4	x	x	x	x	x
5–9	x	–	–	–	–
10–14	x	–	–	–	x
15–19	x	–	–	–	x
20–24	x	–	–	–	x
25–29	x	x	–	–	x
30–34	x	–	–	–	x
35–39	x	–	–	–	x
40–44	–	–	–	–	–
45–49	–	–	–	x	–

SOURCE: Ruzicka and Kane, 1987

mortality among women aged 45–49. Those women who survive to
the age of 50 and beyond have lower death rates than men, in most of
the countries, as is the case elsewhere in the world.

A calculation of the percentage of men and women who survive to
a given age from birth makes a similar point. Figure 1.5 shows this
calculation for Australia and for Bangladesh; as one would expect,
the percentage of Bangladeshis of either sex who survive to any
particular age is much lower than the percentage of Australians but,
from the second year of life onwards, Bangladeshi women of any age
show dramatically lower rates of survival than their menfolk.

VULNERABLE AGES IN HISTORICAL EUROPE

In Europe too, women in the past did not always have a better life
expectation than men, and the amount of female advantage – if
any – could vary quite considerably at different dates, as local
conditions changed.

Figures for Germany (Figure 1.6) suggest that, between 1570 and
1599, a smaller proportion of girls than boys survived at age 15; in the
period 1750–79 the number of women surviving at age 50 was only
just about equal to the number of men at the same age, and between
1630 and 1808 the number of women surviving to age 70 was always
either below, or only equal to, that of men.

Graphs of male and female mortality rates at specific ages in
Britain between 1911 and 1981 show very clearly where there have
been major extra gains for women. Death rates for both sexes, at
each of the four ages shown, have fallen, though they have fallen less
at age 60 than at the younger ages. This is to be expected, of course,
because the most dramatic increases in the expectation of life are
achieved by preventing deaths among infants and small children.
Looking back at Figure 1.1, it is clear that a change from the
U-shaped curve of mortality to a J-curve is the major component of
prolongations in the length of life.

At each separate age in Figure 1.7, however, the pattern is quite
different. Males in Britain have benefited as much as females in
infancy from general improvements in health care and living conditions. Female death rates at age 20 have fallen sharply, as we have
already seen, while the death rates of men have fallen less. The

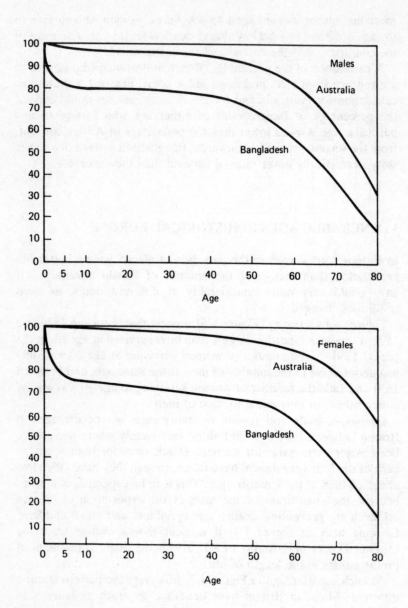

Figure 1.5   Percentage surviving from birth to a given age: Australia 1981/2 and Bangladesh (ICDDRB), 1983.

SOURCE: Australian Government Actuary, 1985, and Shaik et. al., 1985.

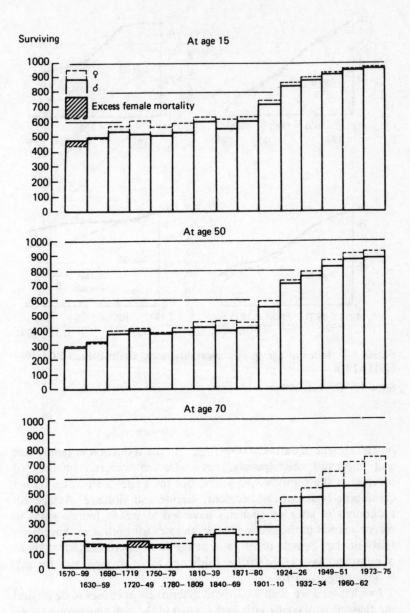

Figure 1.6 Number of 15-, 20-, and 70-year-old survivors per 1000 live births in a selection of parish records, Germany 1570–1975.

SOURCE: Imhof, 1986.

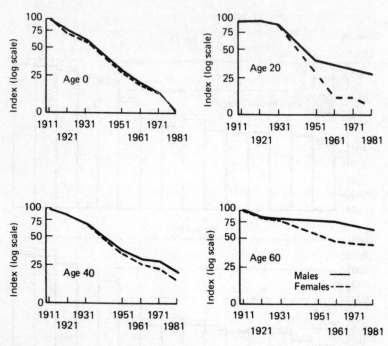

Figure 1.7 Index of age-specific mortality rates, Great Britain 1911–1981 (1911=100).

Source: Daykin, 1986.

postponement of early childbearing, and the reduction in family size and improved child-spacing, have affected women's chances of survival in the reproductive years, but the male death rates reflect continuing high rates of accident, suicide and violence. At age 40, reductions in later pregnancies have led to steady female gains in recent years, but the declines in death rates for both sexes have been fairly similar. Female death rates at age 60 began to fall before those of men, and have fallen further, although there are signs that the gap is beginning to narrow.

In Chapter 2 we shall look more extensively at causes of death and the reasons why young girls and women in the reproductive years do comparatively badly in some countries today, and why they did so in a wide range of countries in the past. At the moment, we are concerned with general trends and patterns of mortality. The two points that concern us here are, *first*, that young girls and women in the reproductive years have traditionally been very vulnerable to death, in a wide range of countries, and that in a few countries they continue to be so, and *second*, that reducing the particular female vulnerability in those age groups has played a very important part in improving women's life expectation, and in improving it relative to the gains men have also achieved.

GAINS FOR BOTH SEXES AT DIFFERENT AGES IN EUROPE

We have already seen that both sexes have increased life expectation in recent decades in most countries of the world. By looking in still greater detail at the age-specific death rates for each sex, we can try to discover some of the other factors which, in addition to changes in female vulnerability at particular ages, have produced improvements in life expectation for one or both sexes. Because most illnesses, as we shall see later, have a particular impact at a particular age, this important point helps to clarify where health interventions have been most successful. Such a calculation also helps to identify how important, in terms of loss of life expectation, are deteriorations in health at particular ages.

A more comprehensive picture of the impact of mortality decline at various ages is provided by Table 1.5. This breaks down changes in life expectation at birth in three European countries into the contributions made by mortality decline at different ages. It also provides some further clues to the widening gap between male and female life expectation in Europe.

Table 1.5 shows that in the Netherlands the additional 4.1 years difference between life expectations of women and men which have been gained over the period between 1950/4 and 1975/8 have largely resulted from the diverging mortality rates above ages 45. Death rates for males aged 45–74 increased during those 25 years, and are shown as a negative contribution of mortality trends to life expectation at birth. As a result, although males in younger age-groups have made reasonable gains, overall male life expectation has risen very little. By contrast, the gains to women's life expectation resulting from mortality declines have increased in each age group above age 14. Among children aged under 15, though, the contribution to total life expectation from declines in death rates has been greater for males: this is because in the past males were more vulnerable to the

TABLE 1.5   *Age components of changing life expectation at birth in selected countries, 1950/54 to 1975/78*

Country	Periods	Sex	Contribution (years) to change in life expectation at birth due to mortality trends at ages								Total increase in life expectation (years)
			0–14	15–24	25–34	35–44	45–54	55–64	65–74	75+	
England & Wales	1950/54 to 1975/78	M	1.37	0.06	0.21	0.20	0.25	0.42	0.24	0.19	3.0
		F	1.16	0.16	0.29	0.21	0.21	0.35	0.64	0.77	4.0
		F–M	−0.21	0.10	0.08	0.01	−0.04	−0.07	0.40	0.58	1.0
Hungary	1950/54 to 1960/64	M	2.83	0.33	0.29	0.30	0.41	0.27	0.18	0.18	4.9
		F	2.50	0.37	0.38	0.29	0.33	0.44	0.42	0.30	5.3
		F–M	−0.33	0.04	0.09	−0.01	−0.08	0.17	0.24	0.12	0.4
	1960/54 to 1975/78	M	1.49	0.08	−0.02	−0.30	−0.54	−0.27	−0.31	−0.12	0.0
		F	1.33	0.07	0.07	0.00	−0.06	−0.01	0.17	0.18	1.8
		F–M	−0.16	−0.01	0.09	0.30	0.48	0.26	0.48	0.30	1.8
Netherlands	1950/54 to 1975/78	M	1.51	0.00	0.15	0.10	−0.05	−0.33	−0.47	0.12	1.0
		F	1.23	0.08	0.16	0.20	0.27	0.55	1.00	1.23	5.1
		F–M	−0.28	0.08	0.01	0.10	0.32	0.88	1.47	1.11	4.1

SOURCE: Lopez, 1984

infectious and parasitic diseases which have now been brought under control.

In other words, in the Netherlands, males in childhood have gained slightly more than females; women aged 15 and over have added years to their life expectation at all ages; but men only between ages 25 and 44. As a result, men in the late 1970s had a life expectation only slightly better than they did in the early 1950s, while women gained 5.1 years over the same period.

Hungary also shows boys achieving an even greater benefit in life expectation than girls from declines in the death rates. Between the early 1960s and the mid-1970s, however, Hungarian men have experienced increased death rates, and decreased life expectation, at all ages above 24.

It seems likely that in other developed countries which show a noticeably increasing gap between the life expectation of men and women, the reason would turn out to be much the same: the failure of adult men to experience the same health gains that women and children have achieved.

England and Wales, however, provide a rather different picture. There has been a much smaller increase in the gap between female and male life expectations, and the increase is largely due to gains made by women over the age of 65. At most other ages, declines in death rates have benefited men more than women. As a result, it has been suggested that women's advantage in life expectation may be beginning to stabilise, or even decrease, if men continue to make slightly higher gains than women in their mortality at middle age.

GAINS TO BOTH SEXES IN SRI LANKA

Sri Lanka is one of those few developing countries for which rather good statistics have been available over quite a long period. As a result, it is possible to look at the contributions which declines in death rates at different ages have made to overall life expectation in this island. The country has made rapid strides in health, which have resulted in increasing life expectation. The figures provide some indication of how those improvements have taken place.

The most striking thing about Table 1.6 is the really remarkable proportion of the total gains in life expectation which have come from reductions in infant and child mortality. In 1945–47, only 78.6 per cent of boys, and 78.1 per cent of girls, survived from birth to five

TABLE 1.6   *Effect of mortality change within a given age range on the increment in life expectation at birth: Sri Lanka, 1945/7 to 1979*

Period	Increment of life expectation at birth (years)	Percentage of total increment accounted for by mortality change within the age range					
		0–5	5–15	15–25	25–45	45–65	65+
Males							
1945/7–50	9.57	34.6	6.3	11.1	22.3	20.4	5.3
1950–54	3.94	44.7	6.7	6.3	15.7	20.6	6.0
1954–67	4.50	83.7	12.3	−1.9	2.2	−3.7	7.4
1967–70/2	0.60	–	–	–	–	–	–
1970/2–79	1.86	63.5	8.4	−3.3	8.9	10.8	11.8
Females							
1945/7–50	10.11	35.0	6.6	13.6	5.4	25.0	14.5
1950–54	4.57	35.8	6.7	8.1	18.9	17.3	13.2
1954–67	7.50	53.4	11.7	6.6	14.0	4.3	10.1
1967–70/2	0.10	–	–	–	–	–	–
1970/2–79	3.21	39.0	7.5	−0.5	16.2	18.1	19.8

SOURCE: Caldwell and Ruzicka, 1985

years of age. By 1979, the percentages were 94.8 and 94.3, respectively. Despite the improvements, the survival of girls still lags behind that of boys.

During the immediate post-war period, 1945/7 to 1950, the gain in life expectation of men and women was equivalent to what had taken half a century to achieve in Western societies (Petersen, 1972). This amazing improvement coincides with the intensive anti-malaria programme carried out in the country. As not much else had changed, it is not surprising that the percentage gain due to reductions in female mortality during the reproductive ages 25–45 was small.

By contrast, in more recent years, women have married and had their babies later, and had smaller families under conditions of improved health care; as a result both the *percentage* and the *absolute* (in terms of years added to life) female gains in the reproductive years has been much above that of males in the same ages. Older women, throughout, seem to have had higher proportionate gains than older men. In other words, while life expectation has risen for both sexes, males have achieved longer life primarily because of reductions in infant and child mortality, while women have made gains not only in infancy and childhood, but also gains throughout adulthood.

Another point which emerges clearly from the table is that the increase in years of life expectation was much larger in the earlier periods than in the later ones. This is partly because it is very much easier to eliminate or control the traditional killers, especially of children (epidemics of infectious diseases, parasites, malaria and so on) than it is to have an impact on the remaining, largely chronic, diseases. That issue is discussed in more detail in the next chapter; the aspect of it with which we are concerned here is that, when one compares the increments to length of life in each period for men and women, those for women have always been larger than, and they have not slowed down to the same extent as, those for men.

A CONTINUING ADVANTAGE FOR WOMEN?

We saw earlier that the gap between male and female life expectation in England and Wales is not quite as large as is the case in a number of other developed countries. There appears to be some doubt about whether women in England and Wales will continue to have the longer expectation of life, or whether the trends for the two sexes are converging. This leads to the next issues:

do the advantages to women tend to widen almost
automatically as life expectation increases, and, in turn,
can we assume that gains in life expectation, for
either sex, are permanent and increasing?

Certainly, the case of Japan suggests a possible future in which the answers to both questions are 'yes'. Around 1950–55, Japanese males had a life expectation at birth of about 62 years; females had an expectation of some 65 years. By 1980–85, life expectation at birth had risen to around 74 years for men and 80 years for women. So far, each year, both sexes show increasing life expectation, and each year, too, the female advantage increases.

However, we have already noted that there is a group of European countries, including the Netherlands, which had rather high life expectation around 1960 but have not made major improvements since – especially for men. These are countries which seem to have got stuck somewhere along the route to extending life expectation, particularly for men.

The experience of males in such countries suggests that while gains in life expectation *may* be permanent, additional gains do not ineluctably continue.

There was also a group of countries, including Hungary, where male life expectation had actually decreased over the period, though that of women continued to improve. Does that mean that women are immune to whatever influences have affected male Hungarians, or just that whatever has caused the decrease among males is taking longer to have an impact on women?

If male and female age-specific death rates for Hungary are examined over a period of time, it quickly becomes apparent that the story is rather complicated. (For both sexes, deaths of those under 5 years of age have fallen steadily, so they have been ignored in Figure 1.8.)

The death rates of those between 5 and 15 have fallen throughout the period, too, but less steadily: in recent years the curve has flattened out, especially for boys. The rates for both men and women aged 15–34 have also flattened out, although at lower levels for women. For men between the ages of 35 and 59, mortality has *increased* by at least 50 per cent between 1966 and 1980 – and 90 per cent of the increase has been concentrated in the ages 45–49. For women, the pattern is similar though less dramatic. Mortality of those aged 40–59 has increased by about 20 per cent over the same period, and a third of the increase is concentrated among women in the five-year age group 45–49. Among the older population, those over age 60, death rates have been rising for men, while they have fallen or, at worst, stagnated for the various age groups of women.

There are various things we can learn from the Hungarian experience. The most obvious one – which nevertheless tends to go against everything we instinctively think – is that *death rates do not automatically just go on getting better and better*, as they have tended to do over the past century or so in the industrialised countries. There is no law which says that health improvements are continuous. In fact, Hungary is not alone in facing this disconcerting lesson: it appears that the USSR, too, has experienced declines in life expectation, though the full statistics have not been made available (Dutton, 1979).

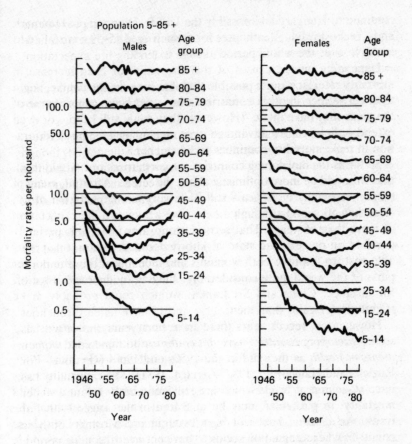

Figure 1.8 Age-specific death rates for males and females aged 5–85+: Hungary, 1946–80.

SOURCE: Compton, 1985.

Neither is Hungary the only country where it is young adult and middle-aged men who are suddenly facing increases in death rates: it is only the farthest along this path. Most of the others are in Eastern Europe, but Portugal has joined the group, as have Norway and Sweden (Lynge, 1984).

Secondly, although women in Hungary have retained much of their health advantage over men, *women are not immune* to whatever changes have caused the problem of declining life expectation. Increases in the mortality rates of middle aged women are, so far,

confined to Hungary and possibly the USSR. However, in Denmark
and Czechoslovakia, death rates for women aged 45–59 have failed to
improve over the whole period 1960–4 to 1979.

Depending on the causes of this stagnation or even increase in
mortality rates, it is quite possible that they may, in due course, begin
to affect women in other countries, who could begin to lose some of
the gains they have made. (However, they could still keep – or even
extend – their *relative* advantage over men as long as the deterioration in male mortality continues to be steeper.)

So far as the developing countries are concerned, one would think
that we could be more optimistic about the future. After all, many of
them – especially in Africa – still have very low expectation of life
(less than 50 years) although others have achieved a life expectation
of more than 65 years. That second group shows that it is perfectly
possible, in our existing state of knowledge and without insupport-
able cost, to improve both women's and men's health in the poorer
parts of the world quite considerably. Judging by the experience of,
for instance, China and Sri Lanka, women could probably make
slightly faster gains than men.

However, in recent years there have been some indications that
*some developing countries have not continued to experience improve-
ments in health* as they did in the 1950s and 1960s (Gwatkin, 1980;
Ruzicka and Hansluwka, 1982; Arriaga, 1981). Their mortality rates
have stagnated at levels which are still quite high. Infant and child
mortality, in particular, may be at a level which suggests that the
traditional diseases have not been brought under control. In those
countries where stagnation seems to have occurred, 'conditions of life
and health are worse for women than for men, putting the former at
even greater risk than the latter in the depressed conditions in which
both live' (Caldwell and Ruzicka, 1985).

SUMMARY AND CONCLUSIONS

Women live longer than men, in general. As we have seen, this
statement holds true both in the wealthier countries of the world,
where the mean life expectation is high, and in the third world
countries where prospective life spans are shorter.

Women have not always been the longer-lived sex, though, and in
a few countries young girls and women in the reproductive ages still

have poorer chances of survival than males. These exceptions are confined to the countries of South Asia – which, however, do contain about 15 per cent of the world's population.

It is usually the case that as life expectation increases, women gain more from that increase than do men. As both sexes acquire additional years of life, women get *more* additional years.

By looking at age-specific death rates at different periods in different societies, it has been possible to see that gains in life expectation do not happen equally across the whole life-span. Reductions in infant and child mortality, and – for women – in risk of death associated with pregnancy and child-bearing, have made the major contributions to improved life expectation.

However, there is no guarantee that all of us – and women in particular – will continue to live longer lives. While the Japanese appear to be doing just that, evidence from other countries suggests that it is quite possible that life expectation for both sexes can stagnate, or even be reduced. Such evidence also indicates that the female advantage may also be reduced in some countries. In other words, women's longer life-span may not necessarily be a permanent, unchanging feature of the future.

There is a considerable amount of variation in the gains to life expectation which have been achieved in different countries, for both sexes, and this suggests that there may be quite complex reasons why women have done better in some societies than others. In the next chapter, some of the explanation for those differences, and for women's general advantage in survival, will be discussed.

2 Explanations for Women's Advantage

The fact that generally women live longer than men could involve a number of explanations for the differences between the sexes. First, it could be that women are generally healthier than men: Graunt in 1662, as we saw, thought that unlikely given the extra health hazards that childbearing posed for women (Graunt, 1975). Or it could be that men and women die of different causes, and that those causes operate rather differently, in particular at different age groups. What Graunt described as men dying 'by reason of their Vices' could be, for example, the excess deaths among males aged 15–24, which are predominantly due to accidents and violence. Or that men are subjected to a number of risks which women are not, or which women suffer to a lesser degree: men may, for example, be more likely to work in a dangerous or polluted environment.

One pair of American commentators on the sex differences in life expectation in the 1950s took the last alternative rather further, and postulated that the difference was due to the exploitation of men by women. (They also, incidentally, dismissed the hazards of reproduction with the description 'this normal but hardly pathological state') After discussing the female advantage in life expectation, they concluded: 'Finally, no doubt, science will come up with something. In the meantime, the American male will continue to pursue the strenuous and the striving life – aided in search of the better things of life by the encouragement of the "little woman" with the placid hormones.' (Vance and Madigan, 1956)

Their assumption was not born out by the research they ultimately undertook, in which they compared mortality of members of Roman Catholic religious orders. Males and females in these orders were assumed to have equivalent risks of the 'cultural stresses and strains of modern life'; when they turned out to have mortality differentials similar to those of the outside world, Madigan concluded that these must have a biological basis (Madigan, 1957). The study was later criticised on the ground that male and female religious orders do not,

29

in fact, have equivalent risks or lack of them: the general verdict has been that the point was not proven.

Alternative explanations imply a mixture of underlying causes – genetic and biological, on the one hand, and behavioural, economic, cultural and environmental on the other.

BIOLOGICAL DIFFERENCES

The biological argument for women's longer mean expectation of life is that there are innate physiological differences in the constitutional resistance to disease between men and women. As the traditional widespread infectious and parasitic diseases, to which everybody was vulnerable to a greater or lesser extent, are controlled, the fact that women do not succumb so easily to the degenerative diseases means that they outlive men.

The biological advantage of females seems to hold broadly true for the animal world. This was shown in a review carried out in the 1940s, which, incidentally, rejoiced in the title 'The role of testicular secretions as induced by the effects of castration in man and by studies of pathological conditions and the short lifespan associated with maleness' (Hamilton, 1948). Its author looked at some 60 studies, carried out on 75 different species representing nematodes, crustaceans, insects, arachnids, reptiles, birds, fish and mammals, and found that in almost every case males had a shorter expectation of life than females of the species. More recent studies have confirmed the general female advantage among animals, but also that there are a fair number of exceptions.

The sex hormones

One explanation which has been put forward for the female biological advantage is the differences in particular sex hormone levels between the sexes. If the womb, male embryos are exposed to high levels of male sex hormones which ensure their full development of male characteristics. It has been suggested that this exposure may lead to higher levels of physical activity, and possibly aggression, during childhood and adolescence – when the excess of male deaths from accidents and violence is particularly high. Levels of male sex hormones increase during puberty, and that increase could also contribute to additional male aggression, but the results of research are inconsistent.

Conversely, naturally occurring, or *endogenous*, female sex hormones are believed to protect women against ischaemic heart disease, which in all cultures seems to have higher rates among men, as we shall see. Most studies of women who have had both ovaries removed have found an increased risk of ischaemic heart disease, and there is also some evidence that early natural menopause similarly increases the risk. However, when men have been given oestrogen therapy, high doses of *exogenous* – synthetic – oestrogen have usually resulted in an increased risk of ischaemic heart disease. And where women have been given postmenopausal oestrogens the results have been confusing: 'it is at present unclear whether postmenopausal oestrogen therapy increases or decreases risk [of ischaemic heart disease], results in no change, or has an effect which varies depending on the specific characteristics of the oestrogens used and the women studied' (Waldron, 1983).

The sex chromosomes

Another theory of biological differences argues that males may be more vulnerable to a number of defects in recessive genes on the X sex chromosome. Men carry a pair of chromosomes made up of one X and one Y chromosome, while women carry two X chromosomes. Because women have a pair of X chromosomes, the 'good' one cancels out the other. But in some animal species males have a matched pair of sex chromosomes, which should theoretically provide the same protection as the human female's XX pair – yet the males still have higher mortality (Comfort, 1979).

Occasionally, a man will be born with an extra Y chromosome (XYY). It has been suggested that further confirmation for a genetic view of male aggression is the finding that men with such an extra Y chromosome are more likely to be found in prisons and mental asylums, but again this remains debatable.

One area where there does seem to be some agreement is that there is a genetic component to the difference between the two sexes with regard to *infectious diseases among infants*. Female babies appear to be less susceptible to these, and this is thought to be connected with immunoregulatory genes carried on the X chromosomes.

So far, it would seem fair to say that the evidence for major genetic contributions to the difference between the survival and life expectation of men and women is rather limited. It is, of course, true that the study of genes has a long way to go, and that the absence of very much evidence to date does not mean that there could not be any more in the future.

BIOSOCIAL DIFFERENCES

Another theory, which blends biology and social pressures, argues that the reproductive roles of men and women have led to social pressure for different behaviour. Because only women can bear and nurse babies, in the vast majority of societies they have been allocated the role of caring for infants and young children. Dangerous tasks have been left to men, and boys have been brought up in such a way as to prepare them for those dangerous (and often aggressive) roles. Thus the cultural evolution of sex roles has been influenced by biological demands.

Such a social differentiation can be applied, for example, to the drinking habits of men and women: in most societies men drink more than women and it has been argued that this is because even occasional drunkenness is detrimental to the care of babies and children, so that women come under heavy social pressure to limit alcohol consumption (Waldron, 1983).

A different variant of the biological and evolutionary approach is the argument that in promiscuous societies or ones in which men have more than one wife, males will have higher death rates than females in the reproductive years because of competition which will lead to aggression between males (Trivers, 1972). Conversely, in societies where each person keeps a single mate, women in the reproductive ages would have higher mortality, because the childbearing demands on them will be higher.

Historical evidence does suggest that in Europe in the past, where marriage to a single partner generally lasted for life, females had higher deaths rates in the reproductive years. Excessive female mortality in those ages, as well as at some younger ages, was a common phenomenon in northern and western Europe before 1920, and even later in eastern and southern Europe (Stolnitz, 1956). The reversal, with men in those ages having higher death rates, has occurred only comparatively recently. In countries like Sri Lanka, the reversal has happened even more recently and swiftly, between the 1950s and 1971. It is unlikely, however, that men's higher risk of death today reflects any changes in marriage behaviour.

The reversals in the relative death rates of men and women have been far too speedy for an evolutionary process to have been involved: evolution in humans, who total only four or so generations a century, is a slow business. There is even debate (Ruzicka, 1986) about whether *any* significant genetic changes have taken place in humans since their early hunter-gatherer days, given that probably not more than some 400 generations separate us from that lifestyle!

There is a certain plausibility to the idea of biological differences creating deep social differentiation, but it is far from providing a complete solution to the greater life expectation of women. For one thing, if the cultural evolution of sex roles had such an overwhelmingly biological basis, it is difficult to see why, in so many societies – including nineteenth-century Britain and the Indian sub-continent today – women and their children have tended to get less, and less varied, food than their men (Ruzicka and Kane, 1985). Under that hypothesis, one would assume that the crucial significance of child-bearing and rearing would be recognised as demanding priority for women in food allocation.

Besides, the theory cannot account for all of the increasing difference between the life expectation between the sexes. Life expectation has risen, in the developed world during the past century, substantially for both sexes but very much more for women: some of the female gain has been from the reduction in maternal deaths, but why should there be a *widening* disparity in mortality from cardiovascular diseases, cancers and motor-vehicle accidents? It seems very implausible to postulate that male aggression and risk-taking have suddenly intensified.

ENVIRONMENT AND BEHAVIOUR

The third, and probably the major, contribution to an explanation of the differences in life expectation between men and women is that they result primarily from different environmental influences and life-styles.

Work

One environmental effect could involve different work-hazards. In some traditional societies only the poorest women do any work outside the home; in most others, women carry out a fairly limited range of activities, largely in agriculture. While in most Western countries, women – especially married women – have joined or re-joined the workforce in increasing numbers since the 1940s, most of them still work in a comparatively small group of industries and occupations. Men are exposed to a wider range of chemical pollutants, industrial and traffic accidents and injuries, and so on.

Cultural behaviour

An example of life-style or behavioural influences which affect the health of both sexes can be found in differing patterns of life expectation in Finland (Lopez, 1984). Although the country is quite small, and differences between urban and rural death rates are also small, life expectation is lower in the east and north than in the south and west. This division is along roughly the same geographic lines as the language division within the country, for the Swedish-speaking people are also in the south and west of the country. Within Sweden itself, male mortality is very low – much lower than in Finland. It appears that the Swedish-speakers share some common patterns of behaviour, across the borders of the two countries, and that these behavioural patterns are different enough from those in the rest of Finland to influence their health significantly for the better.

Life-style and behavioural factors however, may affect the two sexes differently even within any particular community. Different patterns of behaviour are encouraged between the two sexes. Little boys may be allowed or even urged to be more adventurous than girls: to roam unescorted, play with machinery and so on. In England and Wales, there are twice as many road deaths among boys below the age of 15 as among girls of that age group (MacFarlane, 1979). Similarly, when non-traffic accidents are considered, boys aged 5–9 are more likely to die outside the home. Boys are more likely to suffer accidents on farms, or in mines, quarries or factories than girls; presumably they are allowed to play in such places, where a father or elder brother may work, under inadequate supervision (MacFarlane and Fox, 1978). In the river deltas of Matlab, Bangladesh, similarly, twice as many boys aged 5–9 drown as do girls of the same age.

A young man may boost a societally-acceptable self-image through exploiting the power of his car or motorbike: this shows up in the excess male mortality between 15 and 24 from motor accidents. A girl is more likely to boost her self-image by dieting.

As machinery has replaced manual labour, and cars or public transport have become more accessible, the amount of exercise taken by men has fallen. Housework, on the other hand, though less physically demanding than in the past, still involves a healthy amount of physical activity, and most of it still devolves on women. Where households have only one car, the man is often the one who takes it to work, or to a railway station, for the day, while the woman is left to walk to a bus-stop, walk while shopping, walk while taking the baby out.

These are just a few examples of the kinds of way in which culturally accepted roles and behaviour for each sex may influence the health and fitness of each. Another aspect of differential behaviour which is quite often put forward as at least a partial explanation of the difference in death rates is that women are more concerned about their health and more likely to take notice of symptoms, and to do something about them at an early stage, than men. This theory will be discussed in the next chapter, in which we shall begin to examine whether women really have higher reported morbidity rates, and use of health services.

Lifestyle

Lifestyle is closely related to cultural behaviour, of course, but the term is generally used to describe individual behaviour which may differ even within the most similar cultural group. Overall, men may drink more than women – but among men there will be both teetotallers and the three-bottle-a-day types, and there are some women who probably drink more than most men. What you eat, when you go to bed and how many hours sleep you get, whether you take regular exercise – these are the kinds of things that make up your 'lifestyle' and differentiate you from the person next door.

One aspect of individual behaviour has been identified which, by itself, accounts for a great deal of the increase in sex differences in life expectation. It does not, of course, account for all the ways in which males and females have different health profiles – genetic, biological or social. But, for America, it has been estimated that three quarters of the *increase* in the sex differential in life expectation between 1910 and 1962 can be directly attributed to changes in smoking habits. Trends in mortality from heart disease, lung disease and bronchitis, all of which have been causally related to smoking, largely account for different national trends in mortality sex differentials (Lopez, 1984).

CLUES FROM CAUSES OF DEATH

One way to get to grips with each of these various theories is to examine the causes of death for each sex. We can look in more detail at which diseases are the main causes of death, and at how far they vary between men and women. The patterns we find may reflect the different contributions each cause of death makes to the explanation of why women live longer.

For example, in traditional societies the most frequent causes of death are, to this day, infections (especially in childhood) and, in the case of women, conditions associated with pregnancy and childbearing. If female children are less likely to die of infections, some support exists for the theory that they have additional genetic immunity. If women's high death rates are indeed linked to reproduction, a biological contribution is obvious.

Where the pattern is unexpected – in those few countries where young girls have higher death rates than boys, for instance – we may have to look at alternatives, such as whether in such societies girls are treated differently and worse.

We can also make some guesses, based on our findings about causes of death, as to whether existing differences in death rates between the sexes are likely to continue. If the causes are genetic, there is little chance – in the current state of medical knowledge – of change. If, on the other hand, much of the gap between the expectations of life of men and women in the developed world is due to lifestyle differences, such as smoking and drinking, is it likely to continue to increase? Or are there signs that the behaviour of either women or men is changing, and that those changes are reflected, or will result, in a narrowing or widening of the gap in life expectation?

CAUSES OF DEATH: THE TRADITIONAL PATTERN

We can start off by looking at what women die from, and how these causes of death change over time and vary between different societies. We can also see whether, and how far, those causes of death are different from those which kill men. Here, it may be more useful to consider first the causes of death in traditional societies as indicated by some evidence from the developing world. However, two words of caution are needed.

Countries which do not even have a vital registration system to count the total *number* of deaths usually have very poor information on *causes* of death. What there is comes either from small-scale surveys (which may or may not be nationally representative), or from hospital records. In some countries, the very poor (especially in rural areas) may never see the inside of a hospital. In others, only government hospitals are included in the statistics, despite the existence of a large parallel private sector. As a result, many of the data are far from representative. All the same, various broad patterns are evident.

Also, even those developing world countries which still have very high mortality no longer fully represent the traditional picture. Until the 1940s, many such countries continued to have infant mortality rates of over 200 per 1000 births. Today, infant mortality rates of over 100 are thankfully becoming increasingly uncommon. Many infections have been at least partially controlled; a few basic health facilities are increasingly within reach of even the most deprived communities. As a result, data from the developing world today represent, a *transitional*, rather than a completely *traditional* pattern of causes of death.

This second point can be illustrated by some glimpses of the changes which have occurred in China. A survey of causes of death was carried out in part of Yunnan province, China, between 1940 and 1944; I have attempted to reclassify the conditions, which were reported under 27 categories, so that they can be compared with more recent figures. Some categories, like 'convulsions' which accounted for 609 deaths (all but four to children below the age of 14) are impossible to reclassify: that category probably covered neonatal tetanus, and the results of a variety of fevers, as well as epilepsy. The majority of these deaths, however defined, can be attributed to the lack of basic health care, immunisation and sanitation.

Deaths due to *infections and digestive diseases* (dysentery, enteritis and diarrhoea) make up over 60 per cent of all recorded deaths: this is probably an underestimate, as some of the illnesses under 'respiratory' or 'convulsions' were probably due to infections.

TABLE 2.1   *Causes of death, Chen Kung, Yunnan, China 1940/44*

Cause of death	Number male	female	Rank order male	female	Per cent male	female
Infections	1728	1742	1	1	40.6	42.1
Digestive	830	740	2	2	19.5	17.9
Convulsions	321	288	3	4	7.5	7.0
Senility	209	306	6	3	4.9	7.4
Respiratory	223	190	4	5	5.2	4.6
Tuberculosis	223	185	4	6	5.2	4.4
Cardiac-renal	115	132	8	7	2.7	3.2
External causes	117	68	7	9	2.8	1.6
Puerperal fever		93		8		2.2
Infancy	60	64	9	10	2.4	1.5
Cerebrovascular	14	14			0.3	0.3
	3840	3822			90.1	92.2
Ill-defined or unknown	414	314			9.7	7.6
	4254	4136			99.8	99.8

SOURCE: Kane, 1984

There is not a great deal of difference in the causes of death between males and females – partly because the infectious and digestive diseases, and convulsions, affected children most and were at a very high level. Infant mortality alone was probably well over 200 per 1000 live births. Another survey at much the same time in a neighbouring province found that a third of all infant deaths were due to tetanus of the new-born.

Where females survived to bear a child, they might succumb to *puerperal fever*. However, it looks as if, once the reproductive years were passed, women might have had a longer expectation of life than men: there appear to have been more women than men dying of *senility*. Conversely, the males were more likely to die of *external causes* – accidents or violence – or of *tuberculosis*.

The very limited evidence presented in Table 2.1 provides a measure of support for the theory that biological differences affected the survival chances of adult women, and that behavioural differences may have been involved in men's greater susceptibility to death from accidents or violence.

This pattern of causes of death – with a large proportion of deaths concentrated in early childhood, and the majority of deaths due to infections, parasites and polluted water, or faecal-borne organisms, is still common in many developing countries today despite lower mortality rates, and was typical of Europe, too, until a century ago.

EXCESS DEATHS AMONG GIRLS

In the previous chapter, we saw that in some developing countries female children had, or today have, higher death rates than males. The underlying reason for the excess risk of premature female death is usually summed up in the phrase *son-preference*.

Son-preference is recognised throughout the world, but seems to be unusually common in Hindu, Moslem and Chinese societies. It is based on a mixture of economic and cultural values, and is hence one of the cultural or behavioural contributions to sex differentials in chances of survival. Sons, especially in rural families, are valuable because they will eventually work the family land, provide security for parents in old age, and carry on the family name. When they marry they bring an extra pair of hands into the family. Girls, on the other hand, in many societies may not be allowed to work outside the home, and once they are married they are considered lost to their husband's family: thus they have a lower value for parents. Son-preference tends to be most acute where women have low autonomy, limited movement, and little ability to inherit or control property (WHO/UNICEF, 1986).

Some people have argued that the better feeding and care of boys results not so much from discrimination against girls as from an attempt to compensate boys for their biological disadvantage. 'The management of demographic structure by control of the sex ratio . . . results in selective female progenicide to compensate for universally higher male mortality in infancy and childhood' (McKee, 1984).

This theory makes the practice sound rather more respectable than calling it selective neglect of girls, but it is noteworthy that it always seems to be evident in cultures where females have a low intrinsic value. As such 'selective female progenicide' frequency seems to lead to a situation where fewer girls than boys survive infancy and childhood, it also seems a remarkably inaccurate way of achieving a balance of the sexes.

Where son-preference is strong, daughters may be taken off the breast at a younger age, and thus exposed to contaminated or poor quality solid foods earlier in life. The parents may try for another pregnancy more quickly after the birth of a daughter, so depriving the existing girl of breastmilk and of some parental care and attention. The girl will probably get less food than would a boy, and less nutritional food at that. Should the daughter become ill and/or malnourished, she is less likely to be taken to a health facility for treatment; and if she is taken at all it is usually less quickly than would be the case if a boy became ill.

The discrimination is not necessarily most acute in the most poverty-stricken families; indeed, there is some evidence that in some societies differential feeding is more apparent among the richer families in an area. It has been suggested (Ruzicka and Kane, 1987) that this is because in the poorest families there is so little available that everybody suffers; it is only when there is almost enough to go round that it may be distributed unequally. The point here is that a limited reduction in povety will not necessarily, by itself, reduce the discrimination against girls – it has to be accompanied by changes in the status of women.

EXCESS DEATHS AMONG WOMEN

The group of causes of death which affect women alone – those linked with *pregnancy and childbearing* – offer an explanation of sex differentials in mortality due to biological function. This group still has, as we have already seen, enough impact in developing countries for female death rates in the reproductive years to be above those of men of the same age.

Two recent surveys in Bangladesh identify some of those causes of high female mortality (Khan et al 1986; Alauddin, 1986). Both are unusually comprehensive and probably provide a reliable indication of the situation in Bangladesh generally, as well as some insight into the situation in other countries with continuing high maternal death rates.

The first survey – in two areas of rural Bangladesh, see Table 2.2 – recorded 9317 live births and 58 maternal deaths, giving a maternal mortality rate of 62.3 per 10 000 live births, in contrast to less than one per 10 000 in England and Wales in 1984. Maternal deaths accounted for almost half (46 per cent) of all deaths of women aged 15–44, and within this age-range were most common in older women. The maternal mortality rate per 10 000 live births increased to 178 among those aged 35–39, and 250 among those over 40. Only a handful of those who died had been taken to any kind of health centre or hospital when they became ill.

TABLE 2.2   *Most common causes of maternal death in two rural areas of Bangladesh, 1982/83*

Cause	Per cent of deaths
Eclampsia	20.7
Septic abortion	20.7
Postpartum sepsis	10.3
Obstructed labour	10.3
Haemorrhage	10.3
Others	27.7

SOURCE: Khan et al., 1986

The other study, carried out in another rural district in 1982–83, confirms the picture. The maternal mortality rate was 56.6 per 10 000 live births; out of the 48 maternal deaths one in six was abortion-related; the remaining major causes of death were much the same as in the first study; only one woman died in hospital.

Apart from the poor quality of medical care, and the absence of clean – let alone sterile – conditions for childbirth, the surveys indicate high levels of death from haemorrhage. The high numbers of death from induced illegal abortion (almost all the septic abortions had been induced) are also striking.

Those who criticise the provision of contraception in third-world countries, either on the grounds that it is an irrelevance imposed on people with other priorities, or because facilities for careful supervision (particularly of surgical or medical methods) are poor, should consider not only the abortion-related deaths shown here, but the hazards of pregnancy as revealed in surveys such as these, and compare them with the figures given below for European countries.

CAUSES OF DEATH IN COUNTRIES MOVING TO A HIGH LIFE EXPECTATION

Once the traditional infectious, parasitic and respiratory diseases have been brought under control, the list of major causes of death alters quite rapidly. As the China sample in the 1940s provided our

TABLE 2.3 *Changes in the structure and incidence of the ten leading causes of death in the Chinese urban population, 1957 and 1982*

1957		
Cause of death	*Rate**	*%*
D. of respiratory system	120	16.9
Acute contagious diseases	57	7.9
Pulmonary TB	55	7.5
D. of digestive system	52	7.3
Heart diseases	47	6.6
Cerebrovascular diseases	39	5.5
Malignant neoplasms	37	5.2
D. of nervous system	29	4.1
Injuries and poisoning	19	2.7
Other TB	14	2.0
Total		65.7

1982		
Cause of death	*Rate**	*%*
Cerebrovascular diseases	124	22.3
Heart diseases	118	21.1
Malignant neoplasms	116	20.6
D. of respiratory system	48	8.7
D. of digestive system	24	4.4
Injuries	18	3.2
Poisoning	12	2.1
Pulmonary TB	11	2.0
D. of infancy**	51.4	1.6
D. of urinary system	9	1.6
Total		87.6

*   deaths per 100 000 population
** infant deaths per 1000 live births

SOURCE: Liu Zheng, 1986

example of traditional patterns of causes of death (Table 2.1), we shall stay with that country to look at what changes have occurred (Table 2.3). Figures are available for the ten leading causes of death in urban areas in 1957 and in 1982. In 1957 overall Chinese life expectation, for both sexes combined, was 57 years, while in 1981 it was 67.9 years.

By 1957, death rates from the traditional causes had been much reduced in urban areas, but, nevertheless, they head the list of causes, with *respiratory and contagious* diseases and *tuberculosis* responsible for two-fifths of all deaths. In 1982, by contrast, *strokes, heart disease and cancers* – predominantly the diseases of old age – accounted for two-thirds of all deaths: the urban areas of China were rapidly approaching the pattern of causes of deaths found in the industrialised countries of the world. Compare them, for example, with the profiles for North America and Europe in Figure 2.1, and note the contrast with those of Africa and South Asia, for example.

The Chinese figures show the kind of change in causes of death which takes place as countries move from low to high life-expectation. As the statistics are not separated by sex, however, we shall have to move to examples provided in other countries to see what effect changes in causes of death have had on the differences in death rates between men and women.

CAUSES OF DEATH IN COUNTRIES WITH HIGH LIFE-EXPECTATION

We have already seen that in the industrialised countries, there are two periods of life in which women today do much better than men, in terms of death rates. These periods are at ages 15–24, and from middle age onwards.

Excess male deaths at younger ages

The high death rates of young men have been analysed by Lopez (1983), taking the absolute difference between male and female death rates and looking at the specific contribution to it made by different causes. The results are shown graphically in Figure 2.2.

Much of the high male excess mortality which exists in Austria, Portugal, Canada and Australia comes from excess deaths from *motor vehicle accidents*. This is particularly interesting in a case such

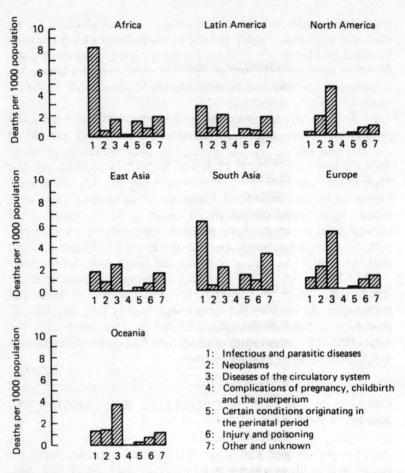

Figure 2.1   Cause specific death rates in UN regions around 1980.

Source: Jakkulinen et. al., 1986.

as Australia, where car ownership and use is virtually universal, because it suggests that the extra deaths are not merely a function of the fact that men are more likely to own and drive a car, as is often true in European countries. Thus the difference in death rates is likely to be one resulting from culturally accepted behaviour, rather than from innate differences in aggression levels, for example. Excess

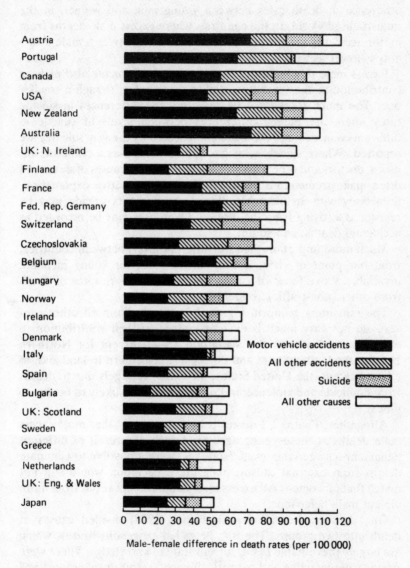

Figure 2.2 Components of excess male mortality at ages 15–44 years : industrialised countries.

Source: Lopez, 1983.

male deaths from traffic accidents are the *major single cause* of the difference in death rates between young men and women in the industrialised world. In the countries where excess male deaths from motor accidents are fewer, the total excess male over female mortality is lower as well.

Excess male deaths from *other accidents and suicide* also make a contribution to the sex differential in death rates, though a smaller one. Too much should not be read into the differences in suicide rates; there are indeed differences between levels of suicide in different countries, but these are complicated by the way suicides are reported. Where suicide is or has been regarded as a crime or sin, juries, doctors and others involved in determining causes of death will often make tremendous efforts to find an alternative explanation. Somebody with an incurable illness who commits suicide may be registered as dying from the disease. Overdoses may be recorded as accidental deaths; and so on.

Much more important than the different levels between countries, from our point of view, is that suicide rates for young men are invariably above those of young women, and so are rates of death from other (non-traffic) accidents.

The remaining group in Figure 2.2 – deaths from all other causes – do not vary much between countries in their contribution to excess male deaths in the age-group 15–44, except for Northern Ireland, the United States and Portugal. In Northern Ireland and, to a lesser extent, the United States, the excess is largely due to deaths from homicide and violence; in Portugal it is more likely to be due to illness.

Altogether, Figure 2.2 makes it extremely clear that most excess male deaths at these young ages are largely the result of different behaviour between the sexes. However, were it possible to eliminate deaths from external causes, male life expectation would still not match that of women. All excess male deaths do not result from more violent male behaviour.

One demographer (Bourgeois–Pichat, 1978) divided causes of death into two groups. The first he called *exogenous* causes, which are largely preventable in the current state of knowledge. These were deaths from infective and parasitic diseases, respiratory diseases and external causes.

The second group he called *endogenous*, and these were deaths from cancers, diseases of the circulatory system, and all other causes. He then calculated mortality from endogenous causes alone, and found that male mortality was higher than female at all ages, and the excess increased markedly with increasing age.

Excess male deaths at older ages

Among people aged 35 to 74, the causes of excess male deaths are very different from those among young men, as Bourgeois–Pichat's calculations would lead us to expect.

Nevertheless, Table 2.4 illustrates very well the assumption put forward earlier that different behaviour between men and women is probably an important reason for women's health advantage. It is true that genetic influences are apparent here – there is a hereditary tendency to *asthma*, for instance. Biological differences are also present: the contribution to excess male mortality made by *cancers* would be 26.2 if the overwhelmingly female mortality from breast cancer did not reduce it by 6.6 percentage points. But the contributions of lifestyle – smoking, drinking, diet, for instance – are all too obvious.

The large contribution to the excess male deaths made by *ischaemic heart disease* nicely illustrates the complexity of underlying

TABLE 2.4   *Average contribution of leading causes of death to the sex mortality differential at ages 35–74 in industrialised countries*

Cause of death		Average contribution (%)
Cardiovascular diseases		48.0
(ischaemic heart disease	38.0)	
Malignant neoplasms		19.6
(lung cancer	14.3)	
Respiratory diseases		10.1
(bronchitis, emphysema, asthma	6.3)	
External violence		10.0
(motor accidents	3.5)	
(other accidents	4.0)	
Cirrhosis of the liver		4.0
Suicide		2.5

Causes and figures in brackets indicate the contribution of specific causes within a classified group

SOURCE: adapted from Lopez, 1983

factors which result in these deaths. Ischaemic heart disease is the narrowing of the arteries carrying blood to the heart, which may result in a coronary thrombosis. It tends to run in families, so that there may be a genetic predisposition to it; there may also be a biological one as it is so much more common among men; it is found among those with high blood pressure, or obesity; but it is also more common in those who take little exercise, have high levels of cholesterol in the blood (linked with high consumption of animal fats) or smoke, and who suffer from stress.

Coronary heart disease in many countries has recently been on the decline as a cause of death. In Australia, for example, the declines have been evident for the past decade and have occurred at a rate of about 3.1 per cent a year for men, and 4.3 per cent for women (Pollard, 1986). Why this has happened remains less clear: people *are* changing their lifestyles – jogging, switching to low-salt and low-cholesterol diets, giving up smoking, have all been quite popular – but at the same time the introduction of coronary bypass surgery has probably prevented many deaths. Why women should have benefited more than men is unknown.

CHANGES IN CAUSES OF DEATH AND CHANGES IN SEX DIFFERENCES

As the gap between male and female life-expectation has widened in so many countries, it is useful to look at some of the main causes of death and see what particular impact each has had on the greater longevity of women.

It has been calculated (Lopez, 1983) that in the industrialised countries as a whole between 1955/9 and 1975/8, *male excess deaths increased* by about 157 deaths per 100 000 population aged 35–74. Over 80 per cent of that increase was due to increased differences by sex in deaths from *heart diseases and lung cancer*.

As can be seen from Table 2.5, much of the rest of the change during the period came from the *increasing female advantage* over men in deaths from *cerebrovascular diseases, genital cancers, and cirrhosis of the liver*.

Men have done better than women in only two areas – mortality rates from *breast cancer* have increased almost everywhere, and almost all those affected are women; and death rates from violence (especially *suicides and accidents* other than motor vehicle accidents) have declined.

The improvement in the incidence of deaths due to non-traffic accidents among males largely reflects improved industrial safety. Changes in suicide deaths are more complicated: the decline in the gap between male and female deaths reflects falling suicide rates for men in some countries, while rates for women remained level or, in other countries, even rose.

TABLE 2.5   *Contribution of various causes of death to the changing sex difference in mortality in industrialised countries at ages 35–74, 1955/9 to 1975/8*

Cause of death	Average contribution of cause to the total change in sex differential	
	per 100 000	*per cent*
All causes	157.3	100
Malignant neoplasms	59.0	37.5
(of lung	39.4	25.0)
(of breast	−7.7	−4.9)
(of genital organs	12.7	8.1)
Cardiovascular diseases	124.0	78.8
(heart diseases	88.1	56.0)
(cerebrovascular	26.5	16.8)
Respiratory diseases	7.0	4.5
Cirrhosis of liver	12.9	8.2
Diabetes mellitus	5.8	3.7
Violence	−4.1	−2.6
(motor accidents	0.4	0.3)
(all other accidents	−4.5	−2.9)
(suicide	−2.9	−1.8)
Senility and ill-defined causes	0.6	0.4

SOURCE: adapted from Lopez, 1983

In the first chapter, we saw that the improvement in female life expectation in the past two decades, compared with that of men, was much greater in some countries than in others.

In the northern and eastern European countries where the gap has widened most, roughly two-thirds of the change is due to the *increased male death rates* from cardiovascular diseases, especially *heart diseases*.

In countries like England and Wales, Australia or the United States, where the gap has not widened much or has even narrowed, the contribution to the differences in death rates from cardiovascular diseases is much smaller. Apart from that, there do not seem to be any common patterns.

PROSPECTS FOR THE FUTURE

In some countries at least, it is possible that the trend towards more male deaths (especially in middle age) will continue for the foreseeable future, and that the female advantage in life expectation will continue to be large and even increasing. However, as we have seen, there is quite a lot of evidence that in many countries the female advantage is beginning to decline, or that women are not experiencing further gains.

There are two ways in which the female advantage in life expectation might not continue to be as great as it is now. With improvements to men's mortality, their life expectation could begin to catch up with that of women. That seems to be perfectly possible: indeed, in some respects the catching up process is already evident.

Where men are gaining

Recent declines in infant mortality – especially in the reduction of deaths from *congenital abnormalities* – have been more *beneficial to males* than females, who already had very low death rates in the developed world. Although the numbers of infants involved are relatively small, the fact that there are more survivors at very young ages has quite an impact on aggregate measures like life expectation at birth.

Stricter controls on drinking and driving, and the introduction of seat-belts, are reducing death rates from *motor accidents* and this, too, should reduce the disproportionate numbers of deaths among young men (Hetzel, 1974). In Australia, for example, it has been estimated that men gained almost a third of a year of life expectation between 1971 and 1981 because of reductions in deaths from motor accidents (Pollard, 1986).

Reductions in cigarette smoking, and improvements in diet and exercise, have already begun to affect male life expectation at the older ages. These behaviour changes have already contributed to declines in male death rates from *coronary heart diseases* in some countries, as we have already noted; they are also beginning to reduce deaths from other diseases of the *circulatory system*, and of the *respiratory system*.

Where women could lose their advantage

Alternatively – or simultaneously – women's health advantage could lessen because women's health may deteriorate. We have seen that in Hungary and possibly the USSR the health of adult women, as reflected in the life expectation at birth and mortality statistics, has actually declined, and that in a number of other countries it seems to have plateaued.

Smoking has increased among women over the past quarter-century, while it has declined in popularity among men. In the past two decades most countries have seen quite considerable increases in the proportion of women (especially married women) who work outside the home. This may expose them to more of those hazards related to work which have typically affected men in the past: *industrial accidents*, greater opportunities for social *drinking*, and so on. Their *stress* levels may also be affected not merely by the workplace, but by the attempt to combine outside work with the pressures of housekeeping and raising a family. As women achieve greater equality with men, too, some of the social pressures to behave in a 'feminine' way – not to drink much, or smoke, or show aggression – are lessening, and with them their protective effect on women's health. However, more recent figures for smoking in America suggest that the current generation of adolescent girls are smoking less (Nathanson, 1984) which suggests that a decline in one social pressure can be counterbalanced by a new one: in this instance, the general anti-smoking drive in the USA.

Most of these changes in women's behaviour are comparatively recent. Deaths from ailments like ischaemic heart disease, or lung cancer, tend to come only after a long exposure to their contributory factors, and hence at older ages: there is little immediate impact. Any increases in death rates of women who have been exposed to these behavioural changes for the past 30 years or so will only be beginning to show up in the mortality statistics towards the end of this century.

In America, increasing female risks, relative to those of men, of *chronic lung diseases* have been linked to changes in smoking habits; and the fact that female death rates from *cerebrovascular* diseases, some *heart* conditions and *accidents* seem to have become resistent to further declines have been noted (Verbrugge, 1980).

However, there is an argument that, even if women's lifestyle changes do affect their health risks, adopting a more 'male' lifestyle is unlikely to have such a dramatic impact as it does in men. One American study (Wingard, 1982), using a sample of 6928 adults in California who were followed up over nine years, tried to assess the impact of 16 demographic and behavioural risk factors commonly thought to affect people's likelihood of death, such as occupation, smoking, weight, sleeping patterns and so on.

Although the study found that the demographic and behavioural factors did affect the risks of death, they did not account for more than a fraction of the overall difference in death rates between males and females. The conclusion was that probably these differences result from a *combination of biological and behavioural factors*, and how these factors interact. In other words, the suspicion is that the whole synergism may interact differently in women from men.

Such a conclusion finds support in the work of at least one French demographer (Pressat, 1981) who writes 'It can indeed be postulated that for biological reasons males derive less benefit from current medical facilities for prevention and care, and hence find it harder to resist natural mortality'. He suggests that the death rates of young males can be improved through the further control of deaths from accidental causes, and from infections, but that the higher male death rates in old age would require not only changes in male behaviour, but new medical and biochemical discoveries to slow down the ageing process.

SUMMARY AND CONCLUSIONS

The more developed countries, with high life-expectation, have reduced the impact of women's major biological health weakness – their reproductive role. Contraception, better maternal health care facilities, and a changed view of desired family size, mean that women are now unlikely to die from causes associated with pregnancy and childbearing.

The processes of 'modernisation' in the poorer countries have also affected people's views about the value of children, especially girls. The number of societies in which son-preference is still so strong that small girls are discriminated against and thus have a greater likelihood of dying is now quite small. As a result, one major cultural threat to women's survival has been reduced. However, in the developing world women's vulnerability to reproductive deaths is still very apparent.

Where these two constraints, biological and cultural, on women have been reduced, it is the worse death rates of men, particularly at ages 15–24 and 35–74, which give women their advantage in life expectation. We can be certain of remarkably few answers to the question of why women generally live longer than men.

There is obviously no single, simple, solution. We cannot just say 'women are born tougher' or 'women have easier lives' or 'women have gentler natures'. There appear to be a number of theories – genetic, biological, cultural and behavioural – to explain the differences in life expectation. While each of them has some validity, it may be that behavioural factors are the most important ones in the more developed countries.

It has already become apparent that a few, specific, causes of death account for a great deal of men's comparatively lower life-expectation. Accidents, especially, have a major impact on the death rates of young men, and one which is potentially avoidable. But there is some evidence that even if these and other avoidable deaths did not happen, women would still live longer than men. Conversely, women's lifestyles may be becoming more like those of men, and women may therefore be facing new risks to their health: risks which could reduce their current advantages in life expectation. Here again, though, there are some indications that the elements in a lifestyle which have such a deleterious impact on men may not affect women so severely.

One reason why it is not easy to understand the advantage in survival which women have is that the causes of death, as we have examined them here, are grouped into very broad categories. In the second half of the book, we shall be breaking down those categories of causes of death – as well as causes of illness – into much more specific conditions. Looking at particular illnesses and detailed causes of death, we may be able to move a little further towards disentangling the basis of some of the sex differences in health.

3 Women and Illness

So far, we have been concentrating on women's health in the context of illness which ends in death. As was pointed out earlier, statistics for deaths are generally better than those for illness, and there is more agreement about what they mean. Defining illness in a population, let alone measuring it, is much more difficult.

WHAT IS ILLNESS?

For one thing, 'illness' seldom means the same thing to two people. We all know people who take to their beds, clutching handfuls of medicines, at the first sign of a cold; we all know others who insist the show must go on, even at the cost of infecting the rest of the cast and collapsing dramatically in mid-performance. Current circumstances may affect an individual's own judgement of health, too. Striving executives have been observed to fall ill at weekends, having firmly shut their minds to symptoms all week. A complaint which might normally send you to bed is less likely to do so if the day in bed means missing your chance of a lifetime to see the Taj Mahal.

Thus health *surveys of self-reported illness*, covering for example the past two weeks (have you taken any medicines? spent one or more days in bed? visited a doctor?) do not necessarily provide an exact picture of ill-health in the community, because they rely upon people's differing perception of their states of health. However, they at least attempt to define 'illness', in terms of taking specific actions to deal with it. Asking people whether they have felt any symptoms of pain or ill-health over a recent period, on the other hand, collects only subjective impressions.

Measures of illness based on such data as *doctor visits*, *medicines prescribed*, or *hospital discharges* are also limited as a source of information on the amount of illness in a community. Whether or not you visit a *doctor* for an illness depends, to a large extent, on individual perceptions of the importance of that illness, and of the costs of a consultation (in time, money and so on), as well as the availability of a doctor. As a result, doctors simultaneously criticise

54

the public for not coming early enough in the course of an illness, and for coming too frequently with 'frivolous' complaints.

Campaigns in recent years to cut down on over-prescribing, particularly of tranquillisers and anti-depressants, indicate the limitations of trying to judge the extent of illness through *prescription rates*. Indeed, as Illych pointed out (1977), the *per capita* use of drugs around the world seems to have little to do with commercial promotion, or anything else, except the numbers of doctors in any particular country.

Hospital referrals again depend first upon the individual seeking help, and secondly on the views of the medical profession – and of the individual practitioner – about the need for further investigation or treatment: they also depend, to some extent, on the availability of hospital staff and facilities. This may result not only in different rates of referral for particular diseases around the country but, where there is an industrial dispute affecting doctors, nurses, physiotherapists or any other hospital personnel, may affect the rates over time.

The definition and treatment of illness also depends on *fashion*, with children's tonsils, for instance, removed in the 1950s almost as a matter of routine, and left, equally routinely, in place today. More importantly, it often depends upon *politics*: judgements about deviations from the 'normal' made by those who control society. This is not only a question of putting dissidents into psychiatric asylums; it surfaces in the assessment of homosexuals as being mentally ill, or in labels like the 'bored/neurotic housewife syndrome'. In parts of the Alps, where goitre was endemic in the last century, those *without* the swelling were laughed at and called 'goose-necks' (Sitwell, 1973). High rates of induced delivery of babies may, when examined closely, reflect the desire of the doctor to avoid weekend or night calls, rather than a risk category of childbirth.

Increasingly, women are claiming that many of the definitions of illness are political ones, in that they have been made by men, and that they are not necessarily valid for women. For example, Durkheim's classical sociological study of suicide (1952) says 'If women kill themselves less often than men, it is because they are much less involved than men in collective existence: thus they feel its influence – good or evil – less strongly'. An alternative hypothesis, writes a female commentator, is that 'the influences women feel are not less strong, but simply different' (Nathanson, 1984).

Such an approach would suggest that we take another look at the causes of illness and death – which may not be the same for men and women. The female advantage in mortality may result, not from lower exposure to the 'risk factors' which men suffer, but to different responses to the same risk factors, or responses to a different set of risk factors altogether.

The recognition that the causes of illness may be different in women also implies a questioning of the diagnoses of those illnesses. During the 1970s, the United States had rates of hysterectomy which were very much higher than those in Australia (which in turn had higher rates than Britain). (Table 3.1)

TABLE 3.1   *Hysterectomies performed in Australia and the United States, 1980*

	Rate per 100 000 females
Australia	232
United States	563

SOURCE: Findlay-Jones, 1986

This did not necessarily imply a different incidence of illness in the three countries. American doctors were describing the operation as good preventive medicine for women who wanted a sterilisation, for example. A certain proportion of women would develop cancer of the cervix or womb, and other gynaecological problems, in later years: so why not have a total hysterectomy now and avoid such a possibility? It is difficult to avoid the judgement that this phenomenon resulted from a highly male-centred view of female anatomy and function. Once childbearing was completed, the womb was viewed as useless, and its removal a simple bit of precautionary medical care.

An alternative explanation, occasionally put forward, was that increased rates of hysterectomy reflected a change in assessing the medical criteria for the operation. Another was the suggestion that the introduction of laparoscopy made possible earlier and more accurate diagnosis of a problem such as cancer. Neither explanation, though, accounts for such large inter-country variation in rates of hysterectomy. In recent years, criticism of these high rates of hysterectomy by feminists and others has resulted in declines in the practice.

All these points have to be borne in mind when we consider the statistical evidence, such as it is, on women's health and illness. There is one further issue, too: many of the surveys on the extent of ill health in a community rely, at least partly, on what is called *proxy reporting*. This means that answers on the health of the family are asked from only one family member, often the wife, as she is assumed to be more easily accessible and probably more aware of family health issues, especially in relation to children. Proxy reporting generally results in under-reporting of the conditions affecting family members other than the one giving the answers. Such conditions may not be known (people do not necessarily describe each headache, or twinge of back pain, to each other), or may not be remembered accurately by the reporter who was not directly affected. Or the condition may be disregarded as minor or irrelevant and thus not reported at all.

However, one thing at least is clear. Health is not merely a matter of being alive. Declines in death rates tell us very little about the overall levels of health – or ill-health – in a community.

A recent French study (Colvez, Robine, et al, 1986) tried to work out male and female expectation of *life without permanent or temporary incapacity*, using French national health surveys to estimate incapacity rates. The results show that in France in 1982, while female life expectation at birth was 8.2 years above that of males, the difference in expectation of life without incapacity was only 5.2 years (Table 3.2). At age 65, the female advantage in life expectation was still 4.2 years, but the difference in expectation of life without incapacity had fallen to 0.8 years; by age 75 there was no difference between the sexes in their expectation of life without incapacity.

Thus the female advantage, in terms of a healthy survivorship, was – except in old age – three years *less* than the apparent advantage shown by the measure of life expectation at birth. In other words, a larger proportion of the longer life-span which women could expect was actually spent in pain or ill-health.

The same study also shows, by sex, the contributions of different types of incapacity to the difference between a life expectation free of disability and overall life expectation at birth. An extra two and half years of *permanent* incapacity which women 'enjoy' over men is the major component of the sex difference in these years of disability.

TABLE 3.2   *Life expectation, and expectation of life without incapacity, at birth:*

	Males years	%	Females years	%	Difference, years
Life expectation without incapacity	61.9	87.6	67.2	85.2	5.3
Temporary incapacity	0.9	1.3	0.9	1.1	0
– with bedrest	(0.3)	(0.4)	(0.4)	(0.4)	(0.1)
Permanent incapacity	7.3	10.3	9.7	12.3	2.4
–housebound	(0.7)	(1.7)	(1.7)	(2.2)	(0.9)
Institution	0.6	0.8	1.1	1.4	0.5
Life expectation at birth	70.7	100	78.9	100	8.2

SOURCE: Colvez, Robine, et al, 1986

When we think of surviving to old age, and how splendid it is that today most of us are likely to do so, we generally have a vision of those later years as being ripe and vigorous. The recognition that much of women's extra life may be endured in permanent suffering is not a pleasant one, and it gives a very different perspective. We shall return to this issue in the chapter on women's health in the later years.

Meanwhile, despite the difficulties involved with definition and measurement, we shall turn to some of the ways in which the health of a community is measured, and see what they can offer in terms of a health profile of women.

HOSPITAL EPISODES

The most recent *Hospital In-Patient Enquiry for England* gives figures for a ten per cent sample of National Health Service patients who were hospitalised in 1984. We shall use this study to look at the difference between the use of hospitals by men and women, because the information is recent and covers a large sample, and is probably fairly typical of the main patterns of differential hospital use in industrialised countries. Very similar patterns can be seen, for example, in the statistics on hospital use in Australia's New South Wales (Yusuf, 1985).

The *Hospital In-Patient Enquiry* provides statistics on discharges from hospital by sex, as well as by diagnosis of illness or death. Unfortunately, the *discharge rates* cover all episodes of in-patient care, whether the patient went home, went to another hospital or institution, or died. Each episode does not mean a new patient; some could have been in and out of hospitals more than once within the same year. This does not particularly matter when it comes to comparing levels of female illness with those of males. More important is the fact that discharges from hospital records cover both *illness and death* together. We already know that men have higher death rates at all ages than women, and therefore we can assume that men's hospital discharge rates will include a larger proportion of deaths, and women's a higher proportion of those who survive to be referred, re-hospitalised or who go home.

Discharge rates

The overall discharge rates for English hospitals are marginally higher for females than for males, at 1015 episodes of in-patient care for every 10 000 males and 1091 episodes for each 10 000 females (Figure 3.1).

As children however, females have lower discharge rates, and they also have lower rates at ages 55 and over. The excess overall female rate is heavily conditioned by the larger number of older women in the population. Even though they show lower rates of illness than men in the same age group over much of their life span, the fact that there are so many more of them surviving to old age results in a slightly higher total rate.

Hospital bed use

Another way to measure use of hospitals is to count the number of *hospital beds used* (Figure 3.2). Females take up fewer hospital beds per million population than males at all ages under 20, and between ages 50 and 74. The higher rate of hospital bed use by women aged 75 and over may reflect the fact that, because women on average marry

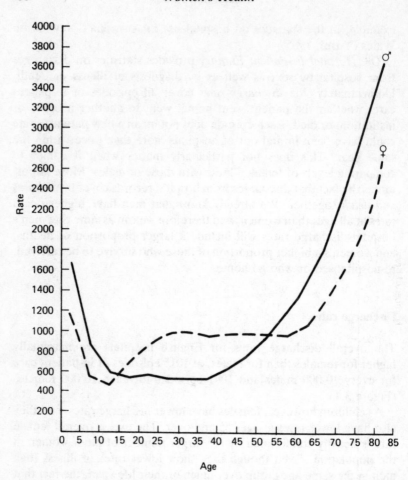

Figure 3.1 Hospital discharge rates per 10000 population: England 1984.
SOURCE: DHSS, 1986.

older men, they are less likely to have a spouse capable of caring for them at home. Indeed, they may no longer have a spouse at all, and they are more likely to live alone: hence, if their illness means that they cannot look after themselves, they are more likely to be put in hospital for general case. The issue of elderly women living alone is discussed further in Chapter 7, on women's health in the later years.

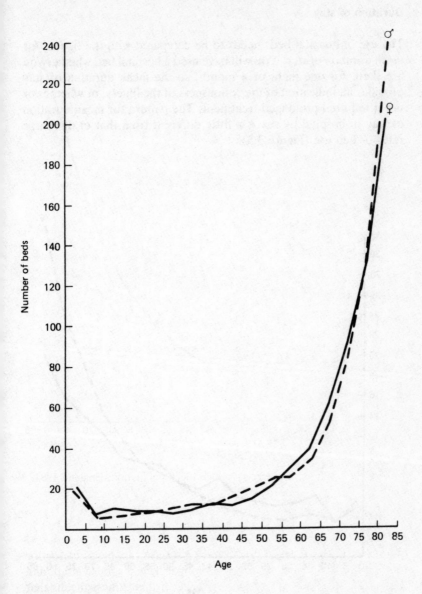

Figure 3.2 Average number of beds used daily per million population: England, 1984

SOURCE: DHSS, 1986.

Duration of stay

The use of hospital beds needs to be compared with the figures for
mean duration of stay. You will have used a hospital bed whether you
are there for one night or a month, so the mean duration of stay
provides an indication of the seriousness of the illness, or whether or
not it required prolonged treatment. The pattern for mean duration
of stay in hospital by sex is a little different from that of discharge
rates or bed use (Figure 3.3).

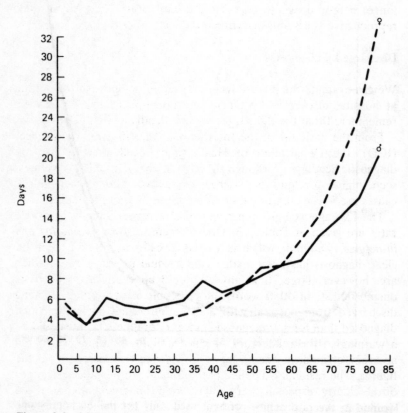

Figure 3.3   Mean duration of stay in hospital, males and females: England,
1984.

Source: DHSS, 1986.

Girls below the age of five have slightly longer hospital stays than do boys, and so do women aged 60 and above. The statistics include deaths as well as other discharges, and small boys have slightly higher death rates, so that more of the hospital episodes of boys may be cut short by death. This may be a contributory factor to the rather small differences in duration of stay between the sexes at young ages. Among the older women, these longer durations of stay may reflect different illnesses, a larger proportion surviving an illness, or different perceptions of how much nursing care men and women are likely to receive at home during convalescence.

In summary, women are less likely to be in-patients in a hospital as children and in late middle age, though they remain in hospital for longer if they do go to one. They occupy more beds during their reproductive years and in extreme old age.

Discharge by diagnosis

We can examine the picture from a different perspective by looking at hospital *discharges by diagnosis*, though here too it must be remembered that the discharges include deaths as well as illness.

From the basic list of the International Classification of Diseases (ICD), the Department of Health and Social Security lists 34 diagnostic headings. Although the total discharge rate is, as we have seen, higher for females, discharge rates for particular diagnostic causes are *lower* for women in all but 13 of 34 those groupings.

The 13 diagnostic groupings which show higher female than male rates are given in Table 3.3. One of them is *signs, symptoms and ill-defined conditions* which is a residual category for use when no clear diagnosis has been made. This residual produces rates which are, however, larger than any of the 33 alternatives in the basic diagnostic list. In other words, more people are described as being discharged from hospital with a condition which has never been diagnosed than for any diagnosed category of illness. That should be a warning to the reader not to place unlimited confidence in the accuracy of medical diagnosis, or in drawing conclusions from the figures. The residual is applied predominantly to hospital discharges of the elderly, especially very elderly, and the larger number of old women in the population probably accounts for the higher female rate.

In terms of rates per 10 000 population, much the most important of these 13 diagnostic groups in which women have higher rates, are

TABLE 3.3   *Hospital discharge rates per 10 000 population, by diagnostic groups showing higher female rates: England, 1984*

Basic list diagnostic group		Males	Females
All diagnoses		1014.7	1090.8
D37	D. of genital system	38.4*	112.8
D38	Abortion		46.3
D39–41	Obstetric causes		12.1
D43	D. of musculoskeletal system and connective tissue	53.2	63.4
D23	D. of eye and adnexa	22.2	27.8
D15–17	Benign and unspecified neoplasms, carcinoma in situ	10.5	26.4
D29	Cerebro-vascular diseases	22.5	24.8
D53	Poisoning and toxic effects	17.3	21.2
D18–19	Endocrine, nutritional and metabolic diseases and immunity disorders	14.6	20.5
D33	D. of oral cavity, salivary glands and jaws	13.6	18.5
D21	Mental disorders	7.3	9.9
D25	Rheumatic fever and rheumatic heart disease	0.9	2.2
D46	Signs, symptoms and ill-defined conditions	143.7	149.0

*includes disorders of the breast

SOURCE: DHSS, 1986

diseases of the *reproductive system*. These are diseases of the female genital organs (including breast), abortions and obstetric causes.

Diseases of the female genital organs is a classification which produces, at 112.8 per 10 000, the highest discharge rate of any group of the 33 defined diagnostic groups on the list: the only other groups of diagnoses with rates anywhere near that are diseases of the respiratory system (males had a rate of 103.7; females 77.4) and of the digestive system (male discharge rate 101.2; female 80.9). These diseases of the female genital system include ailments like pelvic inflammatory disease, menstrual problems, female infertility, and diseases of the urinary system as well as breast disorders.

Abortion in this context covers both spontaneous and induced abortion. The two groups already discussed, together with *obstetric conditions* which covers normal as well as problem deliveries, are clearly ones which are linked to the different biology of the female, and between them they make the major contribution to excess female discharge rates.

Male biological structure does not give rise to an equivalent range of problems: diseases of the male genital system had a discharge rate of 38.4 per 10 000.

In some of the remaining diagnostic groupings in Table 3.3 which show higher female than male rates of hospital discharge, the higher female rate is, when examined more closely, restricted to certain age groups. One, at least, shows the effect which differing life expectation of the sexes has an overall discharge rates: cardiovascular diseases are more common at all ages in men. The overall higher rate for females simply reflects the larger number of women in the older-age population.

A few diagnostic groupings which show higher female than male rates probably result from differences in behaviour. Female children and adult women are more likely to suffer *poisoning and toxic effects*, for example. Small girls, as we shall see, are more likely to be confined to the home than are boys, and in their exploration of the world around them may be tempted to try the taste of household cleaners or jars of pills; boys to climb a tree or cross a dangerous road. Women are more likely than men to attempt suicide by the use of drugs or poisons.

Some of the remaining differences are, however, also linked to the different female biology; *musculo-skeletal* problems being an obvious example. As is discussed in more detail in the chapter on women in the later years, the more rapid deterioration in the bones (*osteoporosis*) of women after menopause than in men of the same age is thought to result from declines in the female hormone levels.

There is another small group of diagnostic classifications of hospital discharges which are supplementary to the ICD basic list, and which are described as *other reasons for contact with the health services*. Women have more than twice as many discharges as men under this heading, with a rate of 38.7 per 10 000 compared with one of 18.2 for men. The difference results largely from differences in contraceptive sterilisation patterns. Most vasectomies are done in clinics or surgeries, as an out-patient procedure, and the male operation is still probably less common. Hence the in-patient discharge rate for male sterilisation is only 1.5, while the female rate of discharge for sterilisation, on the other hand, is 18.7 per 10,000.

The biological basis

What all this suggests is that the major reason that women use hospitals more than men is to do with their different biology. The female reproductive system is more complex, and offers more possibilities for malfunction, than the male one; because it is largely internal it is more difficult to reach for operations such as sterilisation and hence, for a woman, sterilisation may involve a general anaesthetic or other reasons for a hospital stay. Women alone have pregnancies, which may lead to normal childbirth or occasionally involve complications, but which also result in both spontaneous and induced abortions. John Graunt, three hundred years ago, was broadly right when he linked much of excess female illness with reproduction.

In all other causes of hospitalisation, the overall difference in rates between the sexes is comparatively small and can really only be discussed by age. We shall be looking at these small differences in Chapters 5–7.

ILLNESS AS SEEN BY THE FAMILY DOCTOR

As has been pointed out earlier, conditions which reach a hospital are only the tip of the iceberg of ill-health. In many countries it is considerably more difficult, though, to collect information on illness seen by doctors in general practice. Because of the National Health Service, Britain has better opportunities than most countries to gather such data. Three national studies of illness seen and treated in general practice have been carried out in England and Wales, the most recent one in 1981–82 (RCGP et al, 1986, see Table 3.4). Based on a sample of general practices, the third survey recorded both *consultations* – at home or in the surgery – and *completed episodes* of illness.

Consultations

More women than men *consulted* a doctor during the study year (77 as against 65 out of every hundred); for both sexes this was a slight increase over the percentages consulting in the mid-1950s and early 1970s. Women consulted a general practitioner for a somewhat larger number of *episodes* of illness (an average of 2.9 episodes during the year, compared with 2.5 for men). Although there was no difference between the sexes in the number of consultations they had for each episode of illness, the additional episodes meant that the women had more consultations with a doctor during the year (an average of 4 compared with 2.7 for the men).

Diagnostic differences

The more frequent episodes of illness among females show up in the total rates for each category of illness. Males had higher episode rates only for *congenital conditions*, *conditions originating in the perinatal period* (both of which have a very low incidence) and for *accidents*. Some of the excess among women is probably due to the larger proportion of women in the older age groups, where ailments are more common: *musculo-skeletal* problems are one example. However, we shall look more closely at the reported female excess morbidity by age group in later chapters, so here we will concentrate only on the categories which show the greatest disparity.

TABLE 3.4 *Episodes of illness seen by general practitioners: England and Wales 1981/2; rates per 1000 at risk*

Category of condition	Males	Females
Infective and parasitic diseases	123.1	151.8
Neoplasms	11.5	16.6
Endocrine, nutritional and metabolic diseases and immunity disorders	21.5	41.0
D. of blood	3.8	12.4
Mental disorders	67.5	147.0
D. of nervous system	171.0	193.1
D. of circulatory system	99.3	119.7
D. of respiratory system	391.0	423.0
D. of digestive system	78.9	89.3
D. of genito-urinary system	33.0	181.5
Pregnancy, childbirth and puerperium		19.1
D. of skin	126.0	153.8
D. of musculoskeletal system	142.3	191.0
Congenital anomalies	3.3	2.2
Perinatal conditions	0.4	0.2
Symptoms, signs and ill-defined	165.7	235.4
Accidents	138.5	127.9

SOURCE: RCGP et. al., 1986

For the moment, we shall ignore the classification *mental disorders*, which is discussed further on in the chapter. We shall also ignore the residual category of *signs, symptoms and ill-defined conditions*. The most striking differences between males and females are in the rates for *endocrine disorders*, *diseases of the blood*, and *genito-urinary* conditions.

Looking in more detail at the various disorders grouped into the *endocrine* category, it becomes apparent that the one which produces the large difference in relative incidence is obesity. At all ages between 15 and 74, women consult doctors about obesity at least three times as often as men. Over half of the women reported as consulting their GP for any endocrine, nutritional or metabolic condition did so for obesity.

Fashion and, in recent years, widespread publicity about the health dangers of being overweight, may have influenced women to a greater extent than men to seek help with obesity. Most advertising, whether for fitness clinics or for diet regimens, is aimed at, and illustrated by pictures of, women. Alternatively, the doctor may initiate treatment for this condition, when the woman comes to him for contraceptive advice, for instance. It could be argued that women's concern with obesity is good preventive health care, and that their consultations with a GP on this issue are one of the factors which lead, directly or indirectly, to their greater life expectation.

A single condition among those grouped as *disorders of the blood* also accounts for the discrepancy in episodes under that group of diagnoses; it is iron deficiency anaemia. The episode rates for both males and females are very low until age 15; after that the female rate increases rapidly until, in the age group 25–44, it is 20 times that of males. Although the difference is most marked in the reproductive years, it continues throughout adult life, with female episode rates being twice those of men even after age 65.

There have been considerable fluctuations in the patient consulting rates for iron deficiency anaemia over the three surveys, and the report points out that these may reflect people's awareness of their own health, attitudes to visiting a doctor and their ability to treat themselves, more than genuine trends in prevalence. However, it also suggests that the decrease in rates for women – they are now lower than reported in either of the previous two surveys – may be due to a reduction in menstrual problems, associated with a wide-spread use of the Pill. It may also be due to an increasing recognition among doctors (discussed in Chapter 6) that, in industrialised countries, much of the concern about women's lower haemoglobin rates is misplaced. Iron deficiency anaemia is one of the reported conditions, like obesity, which may also reflect a GP's initiative, when a woman comes for contraceptive or pregnancy advice, as much as the woman's perception of her own health.

The third group of diagnoses which show a very high excess of female episode rates are those of disorders of the *genito-urinary* system. We have already seen that the more complex female reproductive system is a major cause of a number of hospital episodes among women, and it is also reflected in their use of GPs. Almost one in four women in the age group 15–44 on the GPs' lists consulted for a condition in this group of diagnoses during the study year. Figure 3.4

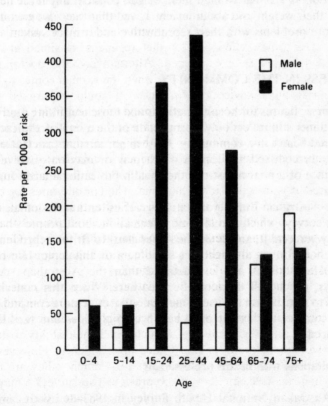

Figure 3.4   GP consultation rates for diseases of the genito-urinary system, by age and sex: England and Wales 1981/2.

shows the very different age pattern by sex of consultations for genito-urinary problems, with the female excess rates being concentrated in the reproductive and menopausal years.

The most common condition in the genito-urinary group, for which both men and women consulted a GP, was cystitis, but there were 14 consultations per 1000 men and 62 per 1000 women. Other common reasons under the genito-urinary heading for women consulting a GP were excess or irregular menstruation, menopausal symptoms and vaginitis.

Biology and behaviour

To sum up, the major differences between the sexes in use of general practitioners are that women seek, or get, considerably more advice about their weight and about anaemia, and that they also encounter far more problems with their reproductive and urinary system.

ILLNESS IN THE COMMUNITY

Of course, figures for hospital patients and those consulting a general practitioner still reflect only a proportion of the overall prevalence of impaired health in a community. Most minor ailments are treated at home, through self-medication which may or may not involve the assistance of a pharmacist or other health professional aside from a doctor.

The Australian Bureau of Statistics carries out a series of national health surveys which reveal some information about people's health as they perceive it, and so do the Americans. In Britain, the General Household Survey also includes some data on this topic. However, the GHS statistics are less detailed than the Australian special surveys, which will therefore be used here. When this material is added to statistics on the use of medical services, a more comprehensive picture of the extent of ill-health among males and females is produced.

Consultations with health professionals

The Australian National Health Survey in 1983–84 asked, among other things, about consultations with all *health professionals* in the two weeks before the survey (ABS, 1986 and 1986a). In addition to hospital and general practitioner consultations, and consultations with dentists, the survey identified a range of other health practitioners, listed in Figure 3.5.

Men are slightly more likely to consult a *physiotherapist* and when the breakdown of these consultations by age is considered, the excess is concentrated in the age group 15–24. This probably reflects the greater proneness of young men to sports-related injuries and accidents. Women appear to be much more likely to consult a *chemist*,

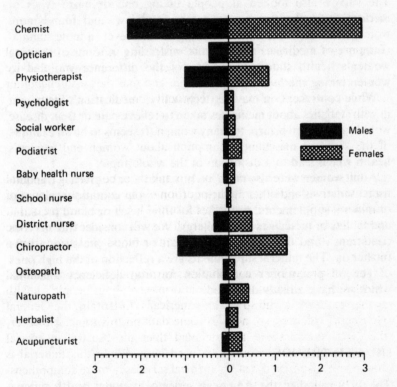

Figure 3.5 Types of other health professionals consulted in two weeks prior to interview: Australia 1983. includes all consultations which took place during the two weeks prior to interview.
Note. Each person may have consulted more than one type and therefore may appear in a number of categories but only once within each category.

Source: ABS, 1986.

but when the age pattern of consultations is taken into account, this turns out to be true only for adult females. Chemists are consulted *on behalf* of more males aged under 15 than females. However, it remains true that females of all ages are more likely to use practitioners of alternative medicine, such as *naturopaths, herbalists and acupuncturists*.

Medication and self-medication

The survey also looked at people taking one or more types of medication in the two weeks before interview, and found more women than men who reported doing so. However, a table summarising use of medicines can be quite misleading in terms of showing women's health status. Four-fifths of the difference was due to women taking the *birth control Pill*!

While contraception may be, technically, 'medication', lumping it in with statistics about medicines taken to relieve pain or treat disease would surely seem bizarre to many women. It seems to be an example of the kinds of masculine assumption about women and women's health which lead to a distortion of the whole topic.

Adult women were also more likely to take – or be given – tranquillisers, sedatives and other medicines for nervous conditions, vitamins or mineral supplements, medicines for their heart or blood pressure, and tablets or medicines for an allergy. We will consider the 'nervous conditions', and the medicines for heart or blood pressure, a little further on. The mineral supplements are a reflection of the high rates of general practitioner consultation for iron deficiency anaemia, which we have already discussed.

HEALTH TRENDS

The 1979 round of the American series of national health surveys shows that women appear to have a particularly high excess in the number of days they spend in bed as the result of illness, in the number of times they visit a doctor, and the number of days on which they report that illness restricted their normal activities (Table 3.5). Information from this survey can be compared with that from earlier rounds, as the American surveys began in 1957. This means that it is possible to use it to look at trends over time, and perhaps explain, or highlight, differences between male and female health (Verbrugge, 1983).

TABLE 3.5   *Health characteristics and the use of medical care services, by sex: United States 1979*

Health characteristics and use of services	Number per 100 persons per year		
	Male	Female	sex ratio
Restricted activity days	824.1	1047.8	0.79
Bed-disability days	334.2	487.3	0.69
Acute conditions	201.5	228.3	0.88
Hospital discharges	14.1	16.5	0.86
Hospital days of care	108.0	123.5	0.87
Physician visits	405.2	537.7	0.75
Dental visits	155.4	183.2	0.85

SOURCE: Rice, 1983

Acute illness

Comparing the 1979 survey with earlier ones, the first trend which is evident is that complaints of acute problems have not generally become more common, but both men and women are more likely to cut down their activities, or go to bed when they suffer, than they were in the past. This probably stems from the fact that it is easier, for a variety of reasons, to take time off than it was in the past; especially time off work.

Short-term disability

Women have always had higher rates for two kinds of short-term disability – restricted ability, and days in bed – than men, but there has been an increase in female rates, especially at ages 45 and upwards, with the result that the difference between the sexes has widened. The difference between men and women has narrowed for the third kind of short-term disability – taking days off work. In the past this was more commonly a male reaction to short-term illness, but women's rates are now catching up, presumably as the pool of employed women has spread, particularly to married women and mothers.

One type of acute disability has risen for both sexes, but more for women than for men, and that is *injury*. The more rapid rise among women, especially those aged 17–44, probably reflects an increasing number of women in the workforce, driving cars regularly, and so on. As women's life styles become more like those of men, they are increasingly vulnerable to the range of injuries which have long been noticed among men. Why male rates should be increasing as well, even if less dramatically, is less easy to answer. Increases in car use and traffic accidents may be a factor.

Chronic illness

For both sexes there has been a rise in the relative numbers of those suffering from a limiting chronic condition, and the rise has been largest in the limitations people find in carrying out their major activities, like jobs and housework. This suggests that people have become less healthy than those surveyed earlier, and that may indeed be true: as death rates decline, there are more people in the population who are in poor health but whose death has been deferred.

However, there are other possible additional reasons for the apparent increase – it may be easier now than it was in the past to change your behaviur or activities because of a chronic condition; and some conditions are diagnosed earlier. Alternatively, increasing health expectations may discourage people from simply accepting a health problem as a normal aspect of ageing: they may expect that, in an age of progress and medical advances, they can be made free of diseases or disabilities.

Woman show the largest increase over time in chronic limiting conditions at ages 45–64. Because men have had higher limitation rates at those ages, women are now 'more similar to men at those ages than before' (Verbrugge, 1983, op. cit.)

FEMALE ILLNESS IN THE DEVELOPING WORLD

Countries which have no reliable information on causes of death are, of course, even less likely to have any about illness in the community.

All one can say is that the high death rates reflect high incidence rates of *infectious and parasitic* diseases, which, like all diseases, affect many more people than they kill. *Malnutrition* is often widespread, especially among women and children. *Respiratory diseases*, including tuberculosis, are also common. So too are *accidents*, though they are often less likely to arise from the use of cars, and more likely to involve burns (from cooking and heating with wood, charcoal or paraffin), industrial accidents where safety levels in factories are poor, and accidents with hoes and other agricultural implements. Women often suffer high levels of *anaemia*, and illnesses related to *pregnancy, childbirth, and the reproductive years*.

Use of services

When it comes to the use of services, the statistics are generally poor. They may also be limited to certain sectors of the population, such as those living in cities, or those using a particular type of health facility or health provider.

However, Thailand, which is a country with a comparatively good health network, and encouraging declines in death rates, also has quite good health service statistics and a series of surveys on the use of health resources. From this material, it is apparent that women use the health facilities in larger numbers than do men (Table 3.6). A considerable proportion of the excess female use can be attributed to the need for pregnancy-related services, but this does not account for all of the differential.

TABLE 3.6   *Medical care services in provincial and municipal health facilities: Thailand 1978*

Out-patients, first visit:	
total number	10 516 274
% male	26.1
% female	36.7
% children under 15	35.2
In-patients:	
total admissions	366 745
%male	22.1
% female: non-delivery	29.5
delivery	21.2
% children under 15	27.2

SOURCE: Porapakkham, 1983

Reported illness

Women are also more likely than men to say they have suffered from some illness during the month before a survey, except in the age group 7–14 (Table 3.7).

TABLE 3.7 *Persons reporting illness within one month of survey, Thailand 1979: rate per 1000 population*

Age	Male	Female	Total	Sex ratio
0–6	438.7	444.1	441.3	98.8
7–14	257.9	239.1	248.6	107.9
15–44	185.3	198.9	192.3	93.1
45–64	235.7	258.5	246.4	91.2
65+	278.3	297.5	288.8	93.5

SOURCE: Porapakkham, 1983.

When the illnesses which were reported were grouped into major and minor ones, rather different sex patterns of reported illness can be seen. Women above the age of 14 are more likely to report minor illnesses; except in the age group 45–64, where women predominate, major illnesses are more likely to be reported by men (Table 3.8).

TABLE 3.8 *Sex ratios (m/f) of persons reporting ill, by age and degree of seriousness of health problem, Thailand, 1979*

Age	Minor illness	Major illness
0–6	97.4	102.9
7–14	108.4	104.6
15–44	88.4	103.7
45–64	94.9	86.4
65+	85.8	111.2

SOURCE: Porapakkham, 1983

Overall, the Thai statistics produce a picture not very different from that in Western countries. They show males in late childhood having a higher likelihood of illness or injury, and adult women reporting more minor episodes of illness and making a greater use of the available services.

PATTERNS OF FEMALE ILLNESS

It is generally believed, or anyhow frequently alleged, that health impairment affects more women than men. Alternatively, it is claimed that they are more likely to notice some health impairment and do something about it. A combination of these assumptions provides one of the common explanations for women's longer survival. It is 'precisely their greater sensitivity to such alarms that makes women more aware of their real or supposed condition, and leads them to find out their precise situation from the doctor . . . . Symptoms of female fragility, beneficial symptoms inasmuch as they probably lead to greater vigilance in regard to prevention and treatment . . .' (Pressat, 1981)

If this were the whole explanation, you would expect there to be no particular relationship between patterns of chronic illness and death. To put it another way, men and women would be likely to suffer similarly from the same illnesses, but men would be more likely to die of those illnesses because women had been treated earlier for their symptoms.

Health care – sought or found?

We have already seen that men have higher death rates for most of the main groups of causes of death. If the lower female rates are due to women doing something about their condition at an earlier stage of the illness, surveys of illness would show equal, or higher, female morbidity from those same conditions that men die of. However, this does not appear to be the case.

The national health surveys in America, for example, indicate that in many instances the sex differences in self-reported activity-limiting conditions are similar to the sex differences in mortality. In other words, men, whose rates of mortality from various diseases are higher, also report more often one of those diseases as limiting their

TABLE 3.9 *Sex mortality and sex morbidity ratios (m/f) for leading causes of death or morbidity: United States 1958–72 (age adjusted)*

Cause of death or illness	Sex ratios	
	mortality	morbidity
Emphysema		4.8
Asthma	4.3	1.4
Bronchitis		1.2
Injuries	2.8	1.5
Heart conditions	1.9	1.3
Malignant neoplasms	1.4	1.0
Hypertension without heart disease	1.3	0.53
Cerebrovascular	1.2	1.6
Diabetes mellitus	0.86	0.83
Arthritis and rheumatism	0.68	0.68

SOURCE: Waldron, 1982

activities. This suggests that women are *not necessarily taking earlier action* to get the diseases recognised and treated and hence protecting their health (Table 3.9).

All of which leaves open the question of whether women take action earlier than men for the *different* diseases which each sex may suffer from.

The Australian health survey found that, at all ages above four years, more males than females reported that they had an illness or condition about which they took no action in the two weeks prior to the survey. The main reason given by both sexes for not taking action was that they did not regard the illness as serious enough to require treatment; it was, however, a reason given by considerably more men than women. (ABS, 1986a)

Rather than the women rushing to a doctor for every sign and symptom, though, the explanation may be – at least in part – that women are far more likely to be screened for, and thus made aware of, a variety of conditions when they visit a doctor for something quite different. Few females, from the time they first seek contraception, can fail to know whether their blood pressure is normal, because it will be measured as a matter of routine before contraceptive options, which include the Pill, are discussed. A young man, on the other hand, visiting a surgery with a sprain or influenza, is much less likely to undergo a blood pressure test.

The fact that many women are routinely screened for blood pressure levels probably accounts for the finding in health surveys that women are more likely to report blood pressure problems, although men have higher death rates from conditions associated with high blood pressure.

A visit for contraception, to a clinic or to many family practitioners, is also likely to involve a gynaecological examination, pap smear, and breast examination. Pregnancy, too, is likely to result in a range of examination which inform the woman of everything from her dental status to whether she is anaemic.

Thus few women avoid being screened for a range of conditions, or being treated if one of those conditions is found. As a result, much of the medication women report taking, and many of the consultations with doctors, may be the result of preventive health initiatives undertaken by the doctors themselves. In such instances, women's alleged 'greater sensitivity to . . . symptoms of female fragility' is beside the point.

However, there are a few discrepancies in Table 3.9 which do suggest that a woman may be quicker to report some symptoms to a doctor. The ratio of male to female deaths from heart conditions is higher than the ratio for heart conditions which were reported to limit a person's major activities. Men have been more than twice as likely to die from *myocardial infarction (coronaries)* than women, but the sex difference in death rates is much lower in *angina pectoris*. This suggests that the sex difference in deaths in the table reflects the larger male rates of myocardial infarction, while the morbidity ratios reflect the higher contribution of angina.

Angina – which results from the gradual narrowing of the arteries – is more likely to be found in men after a coronary attack, but on its own in women; it is also apparently less severe when it is identified in women. So it seems that women may be really more likely to consult a doctor about chest pains (Waldron, 1982).

Do women take more care of themselves?

It has also been suggested that the higher number of acute illnesses, doctor-visits and days of bed-rest which are reported for women may result from it being easier for a housewife to arrange her time – in order to get to a doctor or take a day off – than for an employed man. Such an explanation ignores the increasing proportion of women in the workforce, as well as assuming that both sexes are at similar risk of ill-health. However, a large part of the higher female rates arises from the more complicated female reproductive system.

The American national health surveys show that a quarter of all the sex differences in doctor-visits at ages 15–44 are for *pre-natal care* alone. Studies in other countries have found that about half the sex differences in doctor-visits between adults in middle life is due to *pregnancy and other sex-specific conditions*. We shall find, in later chapters, that the same is true in Britain and Australia, with sex-specific conditions accounting for very large proportions of illnesses and doctor visits, and menstrual problems for days of reported disability.

So far as other conditions are concerned, it does not, in fact, seem to be true that women find it easier than men to get to a doctor. Two American surveys found that women were, if anything, more likely than men to say that problems – inconvenient office hours, the unavailability of a doctor, not having enough time, and so on – deterred them from consulting a doctor (Waldron, 1982).

Among the remaining acute complaints that, in the United States, make up the difference between the sexes in reported morbidity, are *respiratory* conditions and *infective and parasitic* diseases. The statistics from the England and Wales general practitioner survey (Table 3.4) show the same pattern. Infections are also more commonly reported among Australian women (Baghurst, 1986).

This is interesting because male infants have higher death rates for these conditions, and females are thought to have a greater immune resistance to infections; here too it appears that women may be genuinely more likely to identify a complaint and do something about it. But the difference may also reflect different patterns of exposure, with a woman more likely to come into frequent contact with her own and other people's children; and children have the highest rates of infections.

Another contribution to the difference is suggested by the British survey of general practitioner consultations. This found that in 1981–82, urogenital candidiasis (thrush) was the second most common cause of consultations for infectious and parasitic diseases among women of all ages, and the most common cause among women aged 15–44. In previous surveys of GP consultations, carried out in 1955–6 and 1971–72, candidiasis had been sufficiently rare as not to require separate identification. The report of the 1981–82 survey offers no reason for the remarkable increase, but it may be linked to widespread oral contraceptive use. The Pill, like pregnancy, produces changes in the chemical balance of the vagina which make it easier for the fungus to flourish.

Do women have poorer health?

An alternative theory of the higher use by women of medical services is that women really do have a higher incidence of illness. It has been suggested that this is primarily because they have poorer mental health, and partly due to role obligations which interfere with their ability to care for their health. One study (Gove and Hughes, 1979) found that women were more likely than men to say that they were unable to get a good rest when they were really ill, and had to continue to do a number of chores.

This would indicate that while women who are sick may, more often than men, try to cut down their activities or snatch a day in bed, once a man has taken to his bed he is less likely to have to go on coping with the children, or get up to cook dinner, and so on. Women's inability to take sufficient rest when ill because of family responsibilities could leave them vulnerable to a greater frequency of minor illness. When it looked at adults living alone, the same study found that there were few differences in health status by sex, and neither sex reported difficulty in getting rest when ill. Thus it would seem that it is family responsibilities that lead to shorter rest periods when ill, and perhaps a higher frequency of illness itself in women.

There may be some support for this theory from the Australian health survey (ABS, 1986) which found that women were more likely to report short periods of days in bed, but that men were more likely to report having spent 8–14 days in bed.

Women's mental health

It is also argued that women do indeed have more illnesses, because they have a greater incidence of mental health problems. In support of this claim, there are statistics which show that mental problems are experienced significantly more by women than men in most countries. An Australian national health survey showed that women had consulted a doctor for a mental problem almost twice as often as men (ABS, 1979); in England the female rates of mental disorders among hospital in-patients are higher too, as we saw in Table 3.3 earlier in the chapter.

Some of the excess in the total rates reported from the English
hospital survey was caused by the large number of women in the
oldest age-groups. These are the age-groups with the highest incidence of mental disorders, and the disproportionate numbers of
women surviving to those age-groups affects overall rates quite
dramatically. In fact, as Table 3.10 shows, when the figures are
analysed by age and sex the picture is rather different.

TABLE 3.10   *Hospital in-patient discharges and deaths for mental disorders
(D21), by sex: England 1984*

	All ages	0–4	5–14	15–44	Ages 45–64	65–74	75–84	85+
Males	7.3	5.8	4.2	4.3	5.8	12.4	41.6	106.0
Females	9.9	5.5	3.3	3.9	4.4	13.0	48.7	119.8

SOURCE: DHSS, 1986

The higher rates of mental disorder among in-patient females are
limited to the elderly. At all ages below 65, men in fact are more
likely to be hospitalised for a mental condition.

Mental disorders among those hospitalised tend to be severe and
the diagnosis of such disorders may not present too many difficulties.
The issue becomes a lot more complex when we look at mental
disorders in the community, as defined by general practitioners. The
third study of illness in general practice in England and Wales was
clearly disturbed about rates of mental illness reported by those
doctors:

It must be realised that there is considerable variation in the way
that doctors perceive and classify patients by diagnosis. This is
particularly evident in mental disorders, for which the patients
consulting rates in individual practices ranged from 42 to 385 per
1,000 at risk . . ... GPs presumably have different attitudes to the
diagnosis and recording of conditions that are not clearly and
immediately defined by their symptoms (RCGP *et al*, 1986).

Where there are such extraordinary differences in diagnostic rates it is difficult – and even dangerous – to read much into the statistics given in Table 3.11. The old declension 'I am normal, you are eccentric, she is as mad as a March hare' seems to sum it up.

TABLE 3.11   *Episodes of nervous disorders (ICD V) in general practice by seriousness and sex: England and Wales 1981–2; rate per 1000 at risk*

Sex	Category/ condition	All ages	0–4	5–14	15–24	Ages 25–44	45–64	65–74	75+
M	serious	5.4	0.3	0.6	3.3	4.9	7.1	7.9	28.9
F		10.4	0.2	0.8	3.3	7.5	10.4	15.1	48.1
M	inter-	22.1	15.0	8.5	14.1	24.1	34.2	26.8	31.2
F	mediate	50.4	9.2	7.2	41.0	67.9	69.5	60.7	51.4
M	trivial	78.0	191.3	69.5	51.1	60.2	77.4	98.6	106.2
F		88.4	168.8	94.1	79.6	78.4	83.1	85.6	87.3

SOURCE: RCGP et. al., 1986

However, it may be significant that the biggest gaps between the sexes in their rates of mental disorder as perceived by family doctors are in the intermediate, rather than trivial, groups of affected adults. This suggests that whatever the figures do mean, they imply something more than a preponderance of unfulfilled middle-aged women who, it is sometimes said, clutter up doctors surgeries.

The other point of interest is that elderly men – those aged over 65 – seem more often to have mental disorders classified as trivial, whereas women in the same age groups are more likely to be described as having intermediate or serious mental disorders. It is possible that the difference in diagnosis is linked to the presence or absence of family support; elderly men being likely to have younger, fitter wives. or live with other family members, who mitigate or contain their condition.

We can probably assume that a proportion of what are classified as trivial, or intermediate, mental health problems is caused by stress.

The question of whether men or women suffer from more stressful lives or react to the same pressures with differing manifestations of stress is a controversial one, with different studies producing conflicting results that seem to depend as much on the definitions and assumptions of the researchers as anything else.

However, it does seem that social pressures may condition men and women to respond to stress differently: a man is more liable to use violence or alcohol to relieve his feelings (and alcohol may also help him to sleep). Thus men experience higher rates of illness or death from violence – including suicide – and from liver complaints. A woman, for whom such outlets have been traditionally less acceptable, may turn to a doctor for assistance in the form of tranquillisers, anti-depressants or sleeping pills.

Suicide

Women in many societies seem to have higher rates of attempted suicide, although more men actually kill themselves. These differences result partly from differences in the methods of committing suicide which they choose. Women are much less likely to use guns, and more likely to take an overdose. That, in turn, is due partly to the greater chance that they will have potentially lethal drugs around: suicide rates tend to fall when access to such drugs is restricted (Hetzel, 1983). In addition, overdoses of medicines are inherently less liable to a fatal outcome than suicide attempts with guns. They may lead to vomiting, and, besides, their comparatively slow action offers the possibility that the victim may be found before it is too late.

However, for each method of suicide, there are more successful male than female attempts, and this holds true in a variety of countries (Ruzicka, 1968). It seems that women really are more likely to use a suicide attempt as a bid for help.

SUMMARY AND CONCLUSIONS

Given the dubiousness of the diagnoses of mental health, it is difficult to form any conclusions from the figures reported here about women's mental health – or its impairment. A more detailed analysis of the diagnoses which may be stress-related is undertaken in later chapters. Those chapters indicate that the differences in rates of 'mental disorders' may be less significant than they appear.

It would appear that the generalisation about women having more illness, or making use of medical services more frequently, than men needs considerable modification. Much of the excess in hospital use is a function of the larger number of women living to very old age. Women have higher rates of hospitalisation in only just over a third of diagnostic categories, and the most important causes of their extra hospital use are conditions linked with the female reproductive system.

The female reproductive system, together with obesity and anaemia, is also a major contributor to women's excess use of general practitioners. Some of the other conditions reported by general practitioners may have been identified by the doctor when the woman originally visited for contraception or pregnancy. Even taking all this into account, though, it does seem as if women may visit doctors more than men do. We shall examine this issue in more detail, looking at general practitioner consultations by age, as well as sex, in Chapters 5–7.

Women also appear to consult other health practitioners, take more medicines and report more short-term illness, although the pattern varies by age and family circumstance. Again, we shall examine those patterns more specifically in Chapters 5–7.

What is already apparent, though, is that the crude figures examined here need a great deal of qualification. As we saw, the use of the oral contraceptive pill accounted for four-fifths of differential medication between women and men. Hospital beds, and the time of general practitioners, are also occupied for normal healthy pregnancies, and for contraception and sterilisation.

Now, clearly, health administrators need to know how many people, in total, use hospitals each year, or how many consultations a doctor has. The statistics meet the administrator's need. They are not, though, particularly useful when it comes to examining the different health patterns between men and women, because the totals include events which are generally quite irrelevant to the issue.

The use of contraception has nothing to do with being ill. Having a baby is a natural female function and, unless there are complications, it too has nothing to do with being ill. Yet the presented statistics seldom separate out these events, presumably because those who analyse them or use them seldom notice that they are based on a false assumption. The assumption – that taking a pill, or visiting a doctor, implies some health problem – probably does hold true for men. It is patently untrue for women.

Another problem is that women's biological design does seem to be more complicated, and presents greater opportunities for problems, than is the case with men. A considerable proportion of women's use of health services is linked to their reproductive health, or ill-health. It is apparent from the statistics that both the range of conditions affecting men alone, and the numbers of men who suffer from such sex-specific conditions, are very much smaller.

This imbalance in the potential for ill-health is important for several areas of the debate about women's health. If we assume that women are equally vulnerable to all health problems which are common to both sexes, *and* have this extra vulnerability of biological design, then we should indeed be the weaker sex. However, it seems likely from what we have found so far that women are *not* as vulnerable as men to illness which affects both sexes. In which case, we are talking of *genuinely different patterns of health risk* for each sex. That would have considerable implications, not only for comparisons of health trends for the sexes, but perhaps for the provision of services as well.

4 Social and Economic Health Differences

Until this point we have largely concentrated on looking at women's health across societies by comparison with that of men, although we have included trends and patterns of health impairment and mortality of women in the less developed countries to see how far the differences between men and women are universal. In this chapter we shall look in more detail at different groups *within* a society, to see how far health patterns are consistent throughout that society, and try to discover to what extent the differences between men and women which have already been identified apply to all women.

Within any particular country, for example, does women's health differ depending on where they live, or upon family income, or marriage, or some other factor? If all, or most, women have a similar pattern of health and illness, which is different from that of men in the same society, we can assume that these health profiles probably reflect biological differences between the sexes. If all, or most, women do not have a similar pattern of health or illness, the variation should offer further clues about differences in environment and behaviour which affect individual lives and deaths.

One way of differentiating women is through looking at their *social roles*. Are they single, married, widowed or divorced? Do they have dependent children? Do they work outside the home? Each of these conditions separately may affect their health, for better or worse: in combination they may affect it still further, through what is called *synergism*: the combined effect of various factors may add up to more than the sum of the individual effects. In other words, there may be a health impact for a woman in having a job, or of having dependent children. But having a job *and* dependent children may affect her more than either of those two situations in isolation might suggest.

An alternative is to look at women's *social and economic circumstances*, to see whether poverty, or particular types of occupation, increase their health problems. A word of caution is needed here. Where there are differences in health status between groups of women in the same society, it is necessary to be very careful in interpreting them. Phrases like 'poverty' are, in fact, not terribly informative: the question is, what specific aspects of poverty may make for worse health? Is the health problem a result of inadequate or unsuitable nutrition, or of damp or crowded housing, for example – or is it a combination of both? Or – to turn the issue on its head – are some people poor because they have worse health and are therefore unable to earn much?

Often, unfortunately, the fact is that nobody knows what specific aspects of poverty do make the difference. A very important study on inequalities in health in Britain, the Black report (Townsend and Davidson, 1982) concluded that it was difficult to begin to explain the pattern of inequalities 'except by invoking material deprivation as a key concept'; but stressed that it was difficult to pinpoint the exact mechanisms through which that deprivation worked as a cause of poor health.

Poverty is often closely linked with the *environment*. Obviously those living in a slum are very likely to be poor, but in addition, different regions of a country may vary from each other. Some may contain numerous large industrial towns; others are predominantly rural; people living in certain regions of a country may be poorer than those living elsewhere.

None of these conditions influencing people's health are static. They change over time, and when we are considering people's health in relation to them, we have to bear in mind not just current conditions, but those which may have affected people in the past. Health, and health deterioration, are dynamic processes. It often takes a long time for a health impairment to develop, or to produce recognisable symptoms or a full-fledged illness.

WOMEN'S SOCIAL ROLES

Social roles – the ways in which people interact with each other – provide an example of the way conditions may vary over a period of time. For instance, demographic measurements of the number of people born, marrying, and dying at different periods can imply wider cultural changes; changes which affect men's and women's ways of perceiving the world around them and reacting to that world.

The significance of this point may be easier to grasp if we demonstrate it through an example: the well-researched demographic and social history of Germany (Imhof, 1986). Four hundred years ago, less than half of every batch of 1000 children survived to adulthood. Clearly, when infant and child deaths were so common, people may have related to their children in rather a different way, and have had different attitudes to illness or to death.

A maximum of 35–45 per cent of the same cohort of German children survived to marry. Curiously enough, the proportion of married people to the total adult population has not changed nearly so much over time: it has fluctuated at between 70 and 90 per cent. The difference is in the *numbers* of people who live long enough to form part of those proportions.

Changing life courses

A chart (Figure 4.1) shows the changes over time in the life phases of women who married in rural areas of Germany during the past 300 years. The lower diagram shows the division of the whole life course into various segments – menarche, marriage, last birth, menopause, and the 'empty nest' stage when the youngest child reaches age 20 and can leave home. In the two upper diagrams, some of the segments of the women's lives are considered separately – in years, on the left, and as a percentage of expectation of life of women achieving 25 years of age (average age of marriage), on the right.

Traditionally, the average remaining life span of those women who did survive to marry was more or less enough to allow most of them to have their six or seven children and raise three or four of them. By the time the youngest child became self-sufficient, at age 20, the parents were likely to be dead.

Today, women have fewer children, and nearly all of them survive. At the same time, because husband and wife live longer, the average time spent in marriage has increased by about half, from 30 to 45 years. As a result of these two factors, the time spent in childbearing has contracted from about half, to only one-sixth of married life. And, when the youngest child reaches the age of 20, the mother still has about 30 years to live. About 20 years of that time will be spent with her husband. Because women usually marry men older than themselves, and because men die younger, she will spend the remaining 10 years as a widow.

Much of the change in women's life patterns has occurred only in the last hundred years or so. Statistics for Australia (Young, 1989) reinforce that point. Compared with Australian women born in 1860, those born in 1940 had fewer than half the children, and spent only

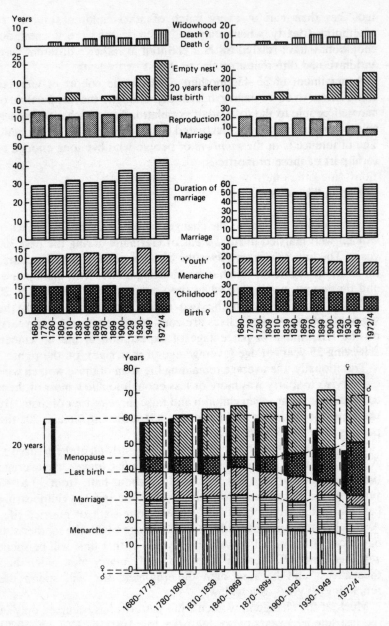

Figure 4.1   Changes over time in the life phases of German women marrying in the last 300 years.

SOURCE: Imhof, 1986.

half the number of years in childbearing and childrearing. Those women born in 1940 had completed their childbearing by the time they were in their early thirties, instead of at around 40 years of age. When the youngest child left home, the 1940s women were 13 years younger than comparable mothers a century ago. They were much more likely to survive their husbands, and, despite being widowed more than ten years later than the women born in the 1860s, could expect to survive alone afterwards for a longer time and to a greater age (Table 4.1).

This extraordinary change in life patterns has all sorts of implications, and offers most women a whole new range of challenges and opportunities.

TABLE 4.1   *Timing of some life-cycle events among various cohorts of Australian women, 1860–1960*

Experience of woman	Birth year of cohort					
	1860	*1880*	*1900*	*1920*	*1940*	*1960*
% never marrying	14	15	13	6	4	increasing
Median age at marriage (years)	24	25	24.4	22.8	21.4	23.2
Av. completed family size	5.1	3.8	2.8	2.9	2.9	
Av. duration of childbearing years	14	11	8	7	7	7*
Av. age at completed child-bearing	40	38	35	33	31	33*
Av. age when last child leaves home	66	64	58	54	52.5	
% ever divorced after 20 years marriage	low	low	low	9	16	
Expectation of life at marriage (years)	44.3	46.7	50.2	54.0	59.3	59.7
% surviving husband	61		69		77	
Av. age at widowhood (years)	56.6		61.8		67	

*Rough estimate. Blanks indicate data not available.
SOURCE: Young, 1989

What is a woman going to do with the 30 years (almost two-fifths of her entire life) which remain once her children have left the nest? Come to that, with childbearing only taking up a few years, and only two or three children to raise, does childbearing alone provide a fulfilling occupation for the first 25 years or so of marriage? What kind of qualities does a woman look for in a partner who is no longer just the co-provider for a family, but who will have to be her sole companion for 20 years after the children have left home? How does she cope with the last ten elderly years as a widow?

These demographic changes are one of the fundamental causes underlying changes in women's perceptions of themselves, their roles and their relationships. But they have another implication as well. In the past, death was a familiar visitor to every family. A baby might live a week, or a month, or a year: equally, it might not. Even if it survived childhood, the time of highest hazard, it could succumb to illness or accident at any stage of life. In addition, there was no way in which disease – in those days, largely contagious disease – could be avoided. Who was struck and succumbed or survived was largely independent of social status, wealth or any other protective measure. Everybody was vulnerable.

There was no single life pattern to which the vast majority of the population conformed; instead, there were a whole series of individual lives, brief, less brief or longer. As life expectation has increased, the amount of individual variation in longevity has decreased. Most of us, once born, can expect to reach our seventies. We, and those who are born in the same period as ourselves, will go to school at the same time, marry within a comparatively short time of each other, have and rear roughly the same number of children, retire at the same age and die within a few years of each other.

As a result, our view of the world has changed. No longer do we see individual lives as brief uncertain visits in the context of infinite immortality. No longer do we assume fatalistically that we cannot intervene to control our lives. The process of secularisation, or modernisation, which has been described, to a varying degree, all over the world, is very closely linked to the amount of confidence we have in our own survival and that of those near to us. Secularisation has probably had even more of an effect on women than on men, if only because it has encouraged them to question their traditional roles and status as wives and mothers – at a time when the demographic rationale for those roles and status has changed almost beyond recognition. Being a wife, and being a mother, mean something quite different today from what our grandparents understood by the term. So when we look at the impact of marriage and children on health, we have to remember that any findings might be very different for people at other periods of history, or in societies with, for example, short lifespans and a different structure of causes of death.

THE IMPACT OF MARRIAGE AND CHILDREN ON HEALTH

Whether or not people are married, and whether they have children, seems to make some striking differences to their reported health status, and these events have a different impact on women to the one on men.

Marriage

The American series of national health surveys, described in the previous chapter, asks the respondents' marital status. Marriage is generally correlated with good health, for both sexes, though it seems to have a greater protective effect on the health of men (Waldron, 1982). Married people report suffering from fewer chronic conditions, fewer days off work and fewer limitations than the non-married, although married women, inevitably, more often report conditions related to pregnancy or reproduction (Verbrugge, 1983).

If it were the case that single people tended to be the less fit members of society, and thus less attractive as marriage partners, then those reported links between marriage and good health would be spurious. However, we find that single women in Britain aged 20–59 have lower age-standardised death rates than married women, at 1.43 compared with 2.23 per 1000 (Whitehead, 1987). That does not suggest that the fittest are being selected into marriage.

Widowhood and divorce

Widowhood or divorce appears to affect the health and survival prospects of men and women rather differently. Because of the age gap between the sexes at marriage, it is more likely that a woman will be widowed than that a man should lose his wife: in England and Wales approximately one in 27 men aged 16 or over is a widower, while the corresponding proportion of women is one in seven (Haskey, 1982).

Women who are widowed survive as well as married women. Men who are widowed, on the other hand, have noticeably worse survival patterns, as can be seen in Figure 4.2. The graphs are based on a study of more than 4000 white adults who became widowed in Maryland, USA, between 1963 and 1974, and who were matched with controls. The study provides a typical example of a well-known phenomenon.

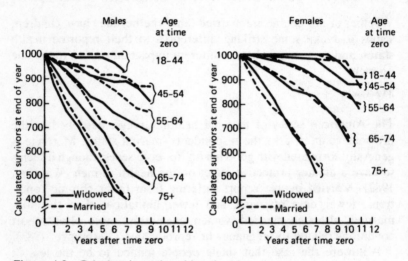

Figure 4.2   Calculated survivorship of widowed and married males and females, by age group and by year after widowhood.

SOURCE: Jeanneret, 1983.

Thus women who are widowed have similar death rates to married women, while widowed men have increased mortality. A similar pattern seems to be true of divorce. A Swedish study looked at divorced men and women who needed various types of hospital care over a three-year period, and calculated the relative risks for the divorced compared with the others (Table 4.2). Divorced men had more than twice as much risk of being treated for infectious diseases, mental disorders and accidents as other men, while the excess risks for divorced women were much lower for almost all categories of diseases.

TABLE 4.2 *Risk ratios of divorced men and women compared to those of other marital status, Gothenburg, Sweden 1969–71: hospital care by main diagnosis*

Diagnosis	Risk ratio	
	male	female
Infective diseases	2.25	1.59
Neoplasms	1.01	1.12
Endocrine, nutritional and metabolic	1.59	1.12
D. of blood	1.91	1.23
Mental disorders	4.50	1.88
D. of nervous system	1.85	1.23
Circulatory system	1.32	1.15
Respiratory system	1.62	1.17
Digestive system	1.35	1.28
Genito-urinary system	1.03	1.34
Pregnancy, delivery, puerperium	–	0.54
Skin diseases	1.58	1.50
Musculo-skeletal	1.59	1.33
Congenital anomalies	1.10	0.03
Symptoms	1.04	1.25
Accidents, poisoning, etc.	2.67	1.42

SOURCE: Nystrom, 1980

All in all, it would seem that the end of a marriage, whether by death of a spouse or by divorce, increases the health risks for men far more dramatically than it does for women, although the reasons for the divergence are not at all clear.

Some of the effects of marital status on health are summed up in Figure 4.3, which shows the excess mortality of males over females by marital status in England and Wales in 1984. (The fluctuations at very young, and very old, ages can be ignored: they result from the very small numbers involved.) The excess is smallest for married men, meaning that their death rates are closest to those of the wives. In other words, women who are single, widowed or divorced fare better than men in similar situations in terms of mortality.

Children

The American health surveys also asked the respondents whether they had children living at home with them. Unfortunately, only

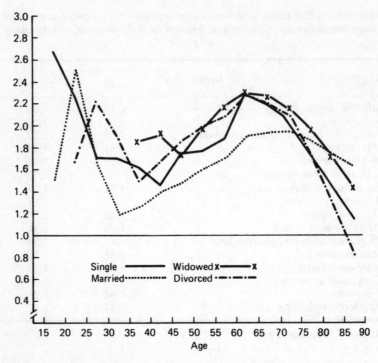

Figure 4.3 Excess mortality of males over females by marital status: England and Wales 1984.

Source: OPCS, 1986d.

women were asked that question, and they were not asked about the ages or numbers of those children, which may well be crucially important when we try to assess the impact of having dependent children on a woman's health. This weakness probably explains the ambiguity of the finding, which was that the presence or absence of children in a household did not seem to have clear links with the health of women.

Inadequate examination of what 'dependent children' really implies may seem surprising. Most women would automatically assume distinctions between levels and types of stress, depending upon whether the dependent children were three pre-school children under your feet all day, or one almost self-sufficient fourteen-year-old. Unfortunately, this naive approach is reflected in much of the literature on differential health, in which there appear to be fairly value-laden assumptions about the roles of housewife and, more crucially, motherhood.

One study, for example (Marcus et al., 1983), considered what it described as the 'fixed role hypothesis' – that people with fewer or more flexible role-obligations were more easily able to 'afford the time' to be ill. The authors defined fixed roles as being the head of the household, making a major contribution to the family income, and having full-time employment. It is probably true that these are more routinely demanding responsibilities than those undertaken by a woman whose children are old enough to take some care of themselves, who may have household help, and who works part-time if at all. But whether such roles are really less flexible than the responsibilities of a woman with two very small children at home, without extended family or other household help, and with a very limited income, is – to say the least – debatable.

In the context of the rather limited definition of 'dependent children', the American surveys found that married housewives with children had better health than the childless. If they were not currently married, mothers had worse health than non-mothers. The stresses and economic constraints of single-parenthood, at least, showed through the survey in poorer maternal health.

JOBS AND HEALTH

Currently-employed men and women show the best health profile in the American health surveys, followed by the unemployed. Those not in the workforce report the worst health. However, men who are not in the workforce are much less healthy than employed ones, while the differences are much smaller for women. In other words, women with some health problems are less likely than men to try to be in, or stay in, the labour force. The findings need to be interpreted with some care, because there is a chicken-and-egg aspect to some of them: for example, a person may be more likely to seek a job if fit than if in poor health, so that the statement that working women have better health than those who stay at home does not necessarily imply that having a job keeps one healthy.

The existence of a job may also affect people's behaviour once they become ill. One study found that whether or not men and women worked was the crucial factor in determining how long they stayed in bed for an illness: on average, those who had jobs were ill for a shorter period. Being employed or unemployed, though, did not explain why women reported more frequent resort to their beds when ill than men in the same category (Marcus et. al. 1983).

MULTIPLE ROLES AND HEALTH

When these two aspects of people's lives – jobs and marriage – are combined, both men and women in the American health surveys show, as one would expect, better health if they are married *and* employed than if they are neither. Among married men, however, those who are not in the labour force have the worst health, followed by those who are unemployed. There was no clear evidence that employed married women with children had better or worse health than those without.

Some studies have found that women with a larger number of role responsibilities use health services, when they do get ill, more often than other women. The explanation generally seems to be that they have fewer opportunities to restrict their activities, and so tend to go straight to a doctor for some intervention to cure them or reduce discomfort (Hibbard and Pope, 1983). They are, effectively, demanding that the health services should enable them to cope, whereas the woman with fewer responsibilities is willing to slow down and rest before deciding to seek treatment. Similarly, the woman with many responsibilities may, when ill, go to bed at least as promptly as one with fewer obligations, in the hope that early treatment will lead to an early recovery.

Employed married women in America have apparently improved in health over time, with those in the 1977/8 survey reporting fewer chronic limitations and better health than did those interviewed in the mid-1960s. By contrast, employed unmarried women have more acute and chronic disabilities than earlier generations, and, after about age 45, more limitation in the kinds of things they can do. Married women who were not in the labour force also reported more chronic conditions and limitations on their activity, especially at the older ages. Thus, middle-aged women with few roles show larger health declines, and middle-aged women who are employed and married show larger health gains.

This finding may come as a surprise: so far we have tended to assume that worsening death rates for women may be a consequence of their lifestyles becoming more like those of men, as more of them take jobs; and of the additional stresses generated by adding a job to family responsibilities.

But if this were true, then we would expect to find that, if anything, the health of working women had deteriorated over the past couple of decades. As more women moved into the workforce, the likelihood that only fittest and most energetic would apply for jobs has declined. This, in turn, means that the health profile of working women would be expected to show more women with some problems. Instead, working women now have a *better* health profile.

This suggests that in some way, active multiple roles have actually improved women's health over time. It may be that working women have gained from increased acceptance and career opportunities, from greater help (mechanical or from the family) with housework, and more support from their husbands. Women who do not work, and do not have husbands, may have lost out in financial support and suffer increasing isolation. It is the worsening health of this group of women with few social roles which has, over the past two or three decades, influenced the overall trends in women's health towards an apparent picture of worsening health.

SOCIAL AND ECONOMIC STATUS AND HEALTH

A common way to look at the links between people's social and economic circumstances and their health is to use their *social class*, as measured by occupation. The occupational categories are used by the British Office of Population, Census and Surveys to determine the social class categories in the following way:

Social Class I	Professional occupations (e.g. doctors and lawyers).
Social Class II	Intermediate occupations (e.g. teachers, managers).
Social Class IIIN	Non-manual skilled occupations (e.g. clerks, shop assistants).
Social Class IIIM	Manual skilled occupations (e.g. bricklayers and underground coalminers).
Social Class IV	Partly skilled occupations (e.g. bus conductors, postmen).
Social Class V	Unskilled occupations (e.g. porters, labourers).
Others	(Armed forces, people with no occupation or no stated occupation, and so on).

Sometimes these divisions are grouped together as non-manual (social classes I to IIIN) and manual (IIIM to V).

As far as health questions are concerned, this classifications has some limitations, as would any other, of course: one important limitation is that it measures a person's *current* occupation. Hence, there is no direct link between occupation and a possible health hazard in the case, for instance, of a man who spent thirty years as an underground miner, but who has now switched to light, semi-skilled or unskilled work after contracting a lung disease.

From our point of view, there is another very serious limitation. Until recently, most studies used the *husband's social class* as the indicator for their wives' social class. In the days when few married women worked, this was probably not much of an issue; but it has become an important one today, when a large proportion of married women work. As a result, it has often been impossible to identify from such studies the real health status of working women by their social class and occupation. Where a clerk has a wife who is a factory worker, for example, their occupational conditions and health risks may be very different.

Women in the workforce

The proportion of women in the workforce in Britain, as elsewhere, has increased remarkably in the past thirty years or so, because of the increased participation of married women. In 1951, less than a quarter of all married women aged 15–59 were economically active: in 1981 almost 60 percent were (Beacham, 1984). What is more, the growth in numbers of economically active women has been most dramatic in the older working ages. Where women previously left the workforce when they had their families, they now return to it, if only to do a part-time job. Some 35 per cent of the female labour force in Britain was in part-time work in 1981, compared with only 3 per cent of the male labour force. The increased number of women who return to work means that more of them may be exposed to any hazards of a particular occupation for a much longer period, and this is another reason for wanting to know women's health status classified by their own occupation.

Women have been, and remain, concentrated in a very narrow range of activities. Almost a third (28 per cent in 1981) of those who work full time are in office work, as clerks, typists, machine operators and secretaries. More than one-third of those with part-time jobs are in domestic labour (cleaners, school helpers) or in the catering trades. Nursing, teaching and sales jobs absorb the bulk of the remaining women who work. Women's more restricted types of activity are probably the reason why, among married women, differences in death rates by social class are less dramatic when they are based on the women's own occupation than that of her husband (Fox, 1982).

Women's deaths by class

Not all women, whatever their biological similarities, are being given the same chances of survival to old age. For Britain as a whole the excess mortality of social classes IV and V compared to classes I and II is 74 per cent for men and, 53 per cent for women. To put it another way, the mortality rates for women in the lowest two socio-economic groups are half as much again as the rates among women in the top two groups.

TABLE 4.3 *Standardised mortality ratios for all causes, by region and sex: Great Britain 1979–80 and 1982–3 (Men aged 20–64 and women aged 20–59)*

Standard region/country*	Men			Women		
	I & II	IV & V	IV & V as % of I & II	I & II	IV & V	IV & V as % of I & II
Great Britain	74	129	174	76	116	153
North	81	152	188	80	136	170
Wales	79	144	182	79	125	158
Scotland	87	157	180	91	141	155
North-West	83	146	176	86	135	157
Yorkshire/ Humberside	79	134	170	78	120	154
West Midlands	75	127	169	77	113	147
South-East	67	112	167	71	100	141
East Midlands	74	122	165	73	110	151
South-West	69	108	156	70	96	137
East Anglia	65	93	143	69	81	117

SOURCE: Whitehead, 1987

*Standardised mortality ratio for all men and all women in Great Britain in 1979–80 and 1982–83 is 100.

The percentage of excess female mortality in classes IV and V over classes I and II varies from 17 in East Anglia, to 70 in the north of England. The variation of the effect of social class on women across the country, though evident from these figures, appears to be *less* than is the case for men: the male excess in social classes IV and V above classes I and II is 43 per cent in East Anglia and 88 per cent in the north.

These are very marked differences, in what is, after all, quite a small country. The lower rates among women of social classes I and II indicate that quite a lot of deaths in the lower social groups could be prevented. Their causes are bound up in some way with the different living standards and general environment within which the poorer women live.

Women's illness by class

When we turn to illness, however, the patterns are rather different. Social class differences in reported long-standing or recent illness are of much greater importance than the differences between men and women. All the same, it is apparent that women of all socio-economic groups are somewhat more likely to report some sort of ill-health. These differences by social class in percentages of those reporting a long-standing illness, or a limiting long-standing illness, and by those reporting restricted activity in two weeks before interview, are shown in Figure 4.4.

Differential behaviour

Differences in socio-economic status do not only imply different work, different living conditions and so on, but also, very often, differences in individual behaviour. One example is cigarette smoking, which, as we have already seen, probably makes an important contribution to a number of early deaths, especially for men. But smoking is itself one of the habits which varies by social class.

Figure 4.5 shows that professional people, as a group, are least likely to smoke, but within that group the proportion of men and women who smoke is similar. Among manual workers, the percentages smoking are much higher, but – especially among the semi-skilled or unskilled – there is a considerably greater gap between male and female levels of smoking.

The figure also shows that cigarette smoking among females is declining far less rapidly than among males, which suggests that in the

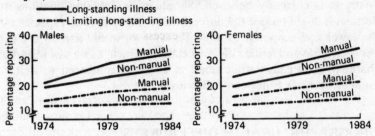

Percentage of males and females reporting long-standing illness and limiting long-standing illness, by whether non-manual or manual socio-economic group: 1974, 1979 and 1984, Great Britain.

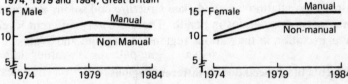

Percentage of persons reporting restricted activity in the 14 days before the interview by sex and whether non-manual or manual socio-economic group: 1974, 1979 and 1984, Great Britain

Figure 4.4 Percentage of males and females reporting various types of incapacity by manual and non-manual socio-economic group: Britain, 1974, 1979 and 1984.

SOURCE: GHS, 1984.

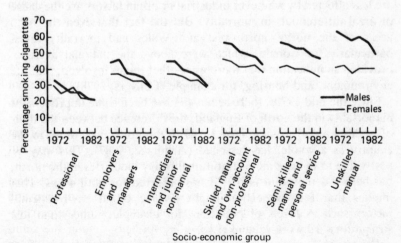

Figure 4.5 Cigarette smoking prevalence, by sex and socio-economic group, 1972–82: Great Britain.

SOURCE: Marsh, 1984.

future some aspects of men's health could improve relative to that of women, if smoking is such an important contributor to ill-health and death as is currently believed. Should male smoking continue to decline, it might reduce the differentials in survival rates especially in the lower soci-economic groups. This in turn would narrow the gap between male and female life expectation, which, as we saw in earlier chapters, is already rather small in England compared to quite a number of other European countries.

GEOGRAPHIC HEALTH DIFFERENCES

Different geographical areas, with their different environment, in-dustries, population, age and class structure and so on, also produce quite marked variations in health. There are very different levels of life expectation in the various regions of England and Wales.

Women's life expectation in different regions

A study of mortality in the mid-1970s (Gardner and Donnan, 1977) found that regions in the south had higher than average life expecta-tion; those in the north, and in Wales, had lower. The range was 3.4 years for men and 2.6 years for women, which suggested that women are less affected by whatever industrial or urban factors are the cause of areal differentials in mortality. But the fact that even the rural areas of the north, north-west and Wales had mortality rates, particularly for women, which were above the national average, provided an indication that there were other things involved, too: the environment, and housing, for example (Chilvers, 1978).

Since the mid-1970s, there seems to have been some improvement in mortality in the north of England: the difference between the rates of both men and women aged 15–44 in the north, and those in the country as a whole, has lessened (Armitage, 1987). This may be partly due to the decline of traditional heavy industries in the north, but here too the point is that it has occurred for both sexes. That implies that the connection might involve broad environmental factors such as levels of pollution, for example, rather than just straightforward work-related risks.

Despite this particular improvement, there has been little overall change in the regional differences in mortality rates for broad age and

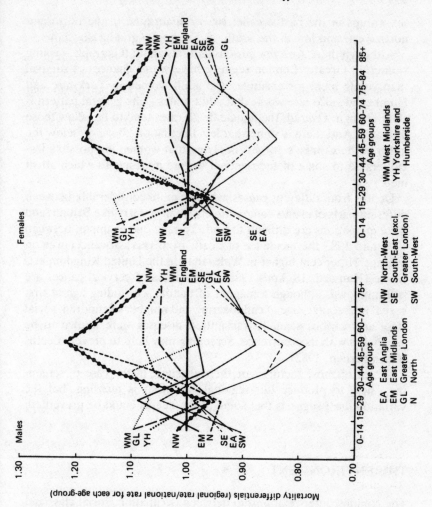

Figure 4.6 Regional mortality patterns for males and females 1982/5: England.

SOURCE: Armitage, 1987.

sex groups in the past decade: rates remain high in the north and north west, and low in the south, as Figure 4.6 graphically shows.

Although there are a few curious features about this graph – young women in Greater London seem to have worse chances of survival than young men, for example, and adult women in Yorkshire and Humberside also fare worse that adult males – the general pattern is clear enough. Overall, the female death rates tend to be below those of males. And there is somewhat less fluctuation above or below the norm in the women's graphs, implying that women are possibly less vulnerable to some of the regional factors in ill-health which affect men.

Deaths from different causes aso vary quite considerably between different parts of even a comparatively small country like Britain, and the explanations are difficult to find. To take one example, between 1979 and 1983 the incidence of death from cervical cancer was on average 11 per cent higher in Wales than in the United Kingdom as a whole (Hansard, 18 April 1985). The causes of cervical cancer are still unknown, although a manner of factors – including age at first sexual intercourse, age at childbearing and number of children, social class and various sexually-transmitted diseases – are known to be associated with its occurrence. Screening may help to prevent deaths (Chamberlain, 1982).

Which of those factors – or their absence, in the case of screening – help to produce this regional variations is puzzling, but the variation itself suggests that some of the deaths could be prevented.

THE ENVIRONMENT

The complex inter-relationship between occupation, social class and environment and their effects on health impairment and mortality shows up clearly in an interesting analysis of the deaths of agricultural workers in Britain during 1979/80 and 1982/3 (McDowall, 1986). More than most industries, perhaps, farming could be said to provide a fairly common environmental framework not only for those who work in it, but for their partners as well.

Admittedly, the category of 'farmer' may range from the wealthy Jaguar-owner whose farming activities are largely concerned with administration and accounts, to the small working farmer whose only help is his or her family. Nevertheless, farmers, farmworkers and their families live in the same countryside, breath the same air, and share a number of common activities. The worker and the farm-owner often use the same machinery and spend much of their time in the open, with the same animals or crops.

Despite this, male farmers aged 20–64 had a standardised mortality ratio of 93, and farmworkers 103, implying that farmers did better than those others who are grouped in social class II, while farm-workers did worse than other workers in class IV. There were also differences between the two groups when the contribution of various causes of death was concerned.

Male farmers, for example, had excess levels of cerebrovascular and hypertensive diseases, and diabetes mellitus, while male farm-workers had excess levels of death from bronchitis. The picture was generally similar for the wives of each group.

The deaths of farmworkers from bronchitis might be linked to the demands of their work, making it difficult for them to retire to bed if they are ill, when there are the cows to get in, or a crop to harvest; such an explanation, however, would not necessarily be valid for their wives. Deaths from bronchitis may also be connected with the notoriously poor housing of this group, and to low living-standards.

Both groups had an excess of deaths from multiple sclerosis, but the excess was much greater among farmworkers. The excess of deaths from multiple sclerosis also showed in the wives of both groups, and in women farmworkers. There is some slight evidence of an association between farming, especially sheep farming, and mul-tiple sclerosis, but what the factor is which influences both those directly working in the industry, and their wives, is unknown.

Both male groups also had excess deaths from *accidents*, and the same was true of women farmers and farmworkers. However, it was not true of the wives of farmers or farmworkers. Accidents, largely due to the use of farm equipment, are obviously a risk which is not encountered to the same extent by the wives of either farmers or farmworkers.

Thus, in a comparatively homogenous industry, defined in only two social classes, we can see indications of occupation-based risks which apply to both classes (leaving the wives unaffected); economic risks (applying to male and female farmworkers and their families); risks from some factor in the total environment (applying to both social classes and both sexes, but – perhaps in combination with other factors – affecting the farmworkers and their wives more severely); and overall class-based risk, resulting from a combination of these and other hazards, which distinguish the farmers from the farm workers and – to some extent – their families as well.

SUMMARY AND CONCLUSIONS

The case of the farmers and farmworkers illustrates how difficult it is to disentangle the various threads which make up the web of health or ill-health that surrounds us all. Except when the cause of illness or death is a major epidemic – which affects most people fairly equally – reactions to a health threat will vary depending on a person's previous health status, their individual circumstances, and the environment they live in. The numbers and kinds of health threat around that person will also be a product of how, where, and with whom, they live. As a result, we cannot draw too many conclusions about the social and economic forces that affect women's health.

We have seen that marriage seems to be beneficial to both sexes, but that men who are married show a greater health advantage than women do. We have seen that many of the studies about the impact of children on a mother's health are flawed by a lack of understanding about what rearing children actually involves at different stages, and that the only plausible finding is that single mothers bringing up a family tend to have greater health problems. Again, though many of the studies are flawed, there seems to be some evidence that women with a full life – work, partners and children – are healthier than those without multiple roles.

The large variations in death rates by women's social class make it obvious that some women face far greater health risks than others. Distressing as these statistics are – because they suggest that many of the deaths among class IV and V women are preventable – it is true that women of all classes still do better than comparable men. Whether it is biological, or reduced exposure to some environmental threats, or a combination of both, there is some protective effect in being a woman. The variation in regional death rates confirms the same point.

However, although the impact of socio-economic class on illness shows up equally strongly, women of all classes report more illness. in each category of ill-health, than their male counterparts. In the remaining chapters, we shall try to find explanations for this paradox by looking in detail at the health problems of women at different ages.

5 Female Health in Childhood

It is in the womb, or *uterus*, that differences in the health, and prospects for survival, of males and females first begin. Some are purely biological, like the numbers of each sex that are conceived and born. Others are genetic, like conditions that are transmitted through, or to, only one sex. But social and economic influences exert themselves, even at these early stages of life, so that it is not always easy to see whether the differences are purely 'natural' or the result of external circumstances. The importance of social and economic conditions increases further once the child is born, and these may override, or even revise the biological advantages or disadvantages that each sex has.

MAKING THE SEXES

Each women is born with a lifetime's supply of eggs, which are stored in the ovary: she never produces more. Actually, she is born with a colossal oversupply, of between 40 000 and 300 000 ova, of which only about a maximum of 500 will ever ripen and be shed. Generally, one ripens in each month and is released to pass down the Fallopian tube to the womb.

There used to be quite a widespread belief that men had a fixed amount of sperm, too, which could be 'used up' through frequent sexual intercourse. Sperm were first seen in the seminal fluid, under a microscope, by a Dutchman Anthony van Leeuwenhoek, in 1677, but it took quite a long time before anybody completely understood what they were or how they worked. Forty years after their discovery, some scientists were still claiming that what they were seeing were microscopic, fully formed, human beings – or, in the case of animal semen, tiny foals riding through the seminal fluid of a horse, for instance (Finch and Green, 1963).

The idea that sperm were a limited commodity which could be used up was one reason that masturbation and *coitus interruptus* were so strongly disapproved of: the man was literally wasting this vital fluid. More importantly, the widespread belief that the sperm were the seeds of life, and that the woman merely incubated them, influenced a view of the sexes in which man was the creator.

In fact, however, sperm are produced almost continuously, in a complicated series of small tubes in the testicles. Hundreds of millions are produced daily, gradually maturing as they move along these tubes and the ductus, *vas deferens*, and then stored in the seminal vesicles which also produce and store the fluid which provides nourishment and protection for them. The whole process leading to a mature sperm takes about three months, and at each orgasm more than 200 million are ejaculated. The length of time it takes sperm to develop, and the way in which they mature, are among the reasons why developing a male contraceptive has proved to be so difficult. Only about one million actually reach the uterus, and perhaps one thousand the Fallopian tubes; only one generally fertilises the egg.

Individual life begins as two cells – germinal cells – one of which is received from each parent. From their fusion all the other cells of the body are produced, by a process of growth and repeated division. In preparation for union, each of the germinal cells has extruded half of its chromosomes, so that each contributes the remaining half to the formation of the cell of a potential new life. Thus both partners share in the creation of the foetus, because the male sperm contributes half of the necessary 46 chromosomes. The other half are contributed from the female egg-cell.

The chromosomes

The basic distinction between males and females comes from those chromosomes. These are the rod-shaped objects, found in the nucleus of every cell, which carry the genes that establish individual characteristics. In humans, there are forty-six chromosomes, arranged in pairs: one pair are the sex chromosomes. The sex chromosomes in females are both shaped like an X; in males there is an X-shaped chromosome and one shaped like a Y. If a sperm with a Y chromosome fertilised the egg (which of course always has an X chromosome), the result will be a male; if it retained an X chromosome, the result will be a female. Hence, the sex of the foetus is dependent on its father.

There have been claims that sperm carrying the Y chromosome have different behaviour to those with an X – and that by taking advantage of this it is possible to select the sex of a foetus. Probably the best-known theory on sex preselection is that of Shettles (1964), who claimed (among other things) that the acid vaginal environment favours the hardy sperm carrying the X chromosome, and that proportionately more sperm with a Y chromosome is produced after a few days' abstinence. Thus, alkaline douches and intercourse following abstinence would help to produce a boy. However, only two very small trials have lent support to this theory, while other research, measuring the ability of X and Y chromosome sperms to move in liquid of varying acidity, has not shown any differences (Kovacs and Waldron, 1986).

Shettles and others also suggested that the timing of intercourse could affect the chances of having a boy or a girl, with some researchers claiming that sex early in the cycle would help produce males, while others argued that males were most likely to be conceived at the time of ovulation. Here too the numbers involved in the early studies were very small, and other researchers have found no significant differences in the numbers of males conceived at different periods of the female cycle.

It seems likely that the claims made for these, and other ways of encouraging the conception of one sex or the other – diet, for example – are based on findings which result from normal, random, variations in the sex ratio. A recent review of sex preselection concluded that 'on the available data there is no worthwhile method of preconceptional sex preselection currently available' (Kovacs and Waldron, 1986). In any case such selection would only affect the chances at fertilisation, and there is evidence that a large number – perhaps even the majority – of fertilised eggs never become implanted in the womb (Research in Reproduction, 1986).

SEX RATIOS

The chances of an implanted egg being male or female are not quite even. Biologists describe the sex ratio at conception as the *primary sex ratio*; they are better at giving it a name than being able to tell us what it is, though. Various estimates of the primary sex ratio have been attempted. The evidence is very limited because it is so difficult to know, in the first few days, that conception has taken place, let alone to find ways of establishing the sex of the tiny embryo.

The estimates suggest that there may be at least 120 male embryos produced for every 100 female. If that is true, it would follow that a larger proportion of males does not survive pregnancy, because, as we shall see, the additional number of boys at birth is much smaller.

Early in a pregnancy – during the first month or so – women are unlikely to know that they are pregnant; it is thus impossible to estimate the frequency of *spontaneous abortions*, let alone identify a sex bias in those pregnancy losses, if any exists. Pregnancy losses during the first month are thought to be very high, but nothing is known about their sex composition.

The picture is no sharper when it comes to sex differences in foetal losses between the second and the sixth month of pregnancy. There have been a larger number of studies to estimate sex ratios, based on abortions or *amniocentesis* (the process of taking some fluid from the amniotic sac surrounding the foetus), but they have produced contradictory or confusing results. At the present time it remains impossible to say whether there are really different risks of loss during the earlier parts of pregnancy, or whether any possible sex differences in risk may vary at different periods of the pregnancy, or in different genetic populations.

However, things become much clearer when one looks at *stillbirths*, or late foetal deaths from the seventh month of pregnancy onwards. It seems that, in the developed countries over the course of this century, there has been a change in the pattern of late foetal deaths. Late foetal mortality was higher for males than for females in the early 1900s, but the difference between the sexes has either narrowed considerably, or disappeared, in recent years. From a sample of births registered in Western Europe between 1929 and 1937, the stillbirth sex ratio was 126.7; the stillbirth ratio in the United States based on births between 1941 and 1945 was 124.1 (Tietze, 1978). In England and Wales in 1983 it was 111.1.

The reason for the reduction in sex ratios of stillborn babies is that males are more likely to suffer a death due to difficult labour, birth injuries, or to the diseases or accidents of the mother. Females suffer stillbirths primarily because of *congenital malformations*. With better maternal health and obstetric care, the porportion of stillbirths due to difficult labour, birth injuries and the mother's health has fallen, and with it the male stillbirth rate. Thus, at this stage of pregnancy at least, the ratio of male to female deaths depends not only on biological and genital factors, but also on the environmental ones of maternal health and obstetric care.

The *secondary sex ratio*, or the sex ratio at live birth, is usually around 104–6 males to every 100 females. There is still some argument about whether that ratio holds true throughout the world. In China and some other South Asian populations, the sex ratio seems to be slightly higher – 106 or a little above – and in Africa rather lower.

It is difficult to establish whether these are genuine differences or not, because many developing countries do not have any effective system of registering births, and few of those births take place in a hospital or with a medical attendant. Even where there is a registration system, people may not bother to record a birth which is followed fairly shortly by the death of the baby. So the estimates of sex ratio at birth may be based on samples or other small numbers (for example, of births taking place in a hospital) where random variations can give a distorted picture: there need to be a very large number of births in order to calculate a reliable sex ratio.

Alternatively, if parents only get around to registering a child who looks like surviving, reported sex ratios may be based on infants who have lived through their first week, or month. Boy babies, like male foetuses, are more vulnerable than female ones, so that the ratio of survivors is likely to be lower than the sex ratio at birth. On the other hand, in a few countries where girl children are less valued than males, their survival chances are lower – and, even when they do survive, their parents are less likely to register their birth. All the same, there are indications – like the lower sex ratio of about 103 among black Americans – that there may be real, though small, genetic variations in the sex ratio at birth (Stern, 1973).

GENETIC DISORDERS

It is not only the sex of an embryo which is decided when a particular sperm joins with an egg and the fertilised egg is implanted in the womb. Every chromosome carries numerous genes, which will determine the characteristics of the child. Some of these genetic characteristics are described as *dominant* – brown eyes, for example – others as *recessive* (blue eyes). Each has an equal tendency to be transmitted. Where an individual gets a similar genetic characteristic, regardless of whether it is dominant or recessive, from both parents, that individual will reproduce that characteristic. With genes for blue eyes from both parents, the result will be a blue-eyed child. However, if the genetic characteristics received from each parent are different, the dominant one will be reproduced. If one parent transmits the genes for blue eyes and the other the genes for brown, the child will have brown eyes.

Both the chromosomes transmitted by each parent, and the genes on those chromosomes, have the potential to transmit disorders, like any other characteristic carried by those parents. Disorders which are carried on a single gene are described as *dominant, recessive or sex-linked*. They may affect up to one in 100 births.

All those born with a condition due to a dominant gene will develop that condition. There is, in turn, a 50 per cent chance that any child they produce will inherit it. Huntington's chorea is an example of a disorder carried on a dominant gene. Where the gene is recessive, like the one which carries cystic fibrosis, it is unlikely to be passed on unless both parents carry such a gene: in which case each child would have a 25 per cent chance of inheriting it.

Sex-linked genetic disorders are transmitted through the pair of chromosomes which establish sex. Conditions carried by the genes on the sex chromosomes are the ones which affect males and females differently. Sex chromosome abnormalities occur twice as frequently in males as in females, and they become more common where the mother is older.

There are genes on the X chromosome which influence various traits which can lead to recessive disorders. The reason why these particular sex-linked genetic disorders are less common among females is that females have two X chromosomes. This means that if one carries the gene for an X-linked recessive disorder, the protective effects of a normal gene on the other X chromosome will usually cancel out its impact. Because males have only one X chromosome, though, the genetic disorder is much more liable to occur.

Colour-blindness is an example of one recessive genetic disorder which – in one or other of its manifestations – is very common, being found in about one person in 50. It is roughly 20 times more common in men than in women. Because the condition is due to a recessive gene on the X chromosome, a female would have to inherit it from both parents to be affected. All her sons would be likewise affected. If only one of her X chromosomes carried the trait, however, she would not be colour-blind but her sons would have a 50 per cent chance of being so. In either case, a colour-blind son would not transmit the disease in turn to his sons, since they would inherit only his Y sex chromosome.

Haemophilia (heavy bleeding after even a slight wound) is probably the best-known example of a sex-selective hereditary illness, although it is comparatively rare: being found among probably only one in 3000 to 4000 births in the European races, where it is most frequent. Although transmitted by females, on the X chromosome, it is almost entirely confined to men, affecting 50 per cent of sons and leaving 50 per cent of daughters as carriers.

The X sex chromosome also carries a variety of additional genes which influence the functioning of the body's *immune system*. Here again, males are more vulnerable to any defective gene since they do not have a second X chromosome to counterbalance it. This is thought to be why female infants in the majority of countries around the world tend to have lower death rates from *infectious diseases* (Waldron, 1983). Those specific X-linked immunodeficiency syndromes which have been identified so far are comparatively rare, but it is believed that there may be other, more common ones which, however, are less easy to identify because they may only slightly reduce the functioning of the immune system.

Chromosomes may, in addition, create a health threat in the embryo through their own malfunction. *Chromosome abnormalities* are found in only about 0.2 per cent of live births (Table 5.1). They are divided into two types – abnormalities of the sex chromosomes, and where an autosomal (an extra, single) chromosome is produced. Down's syndrome is the most common example of the latter group,

TABLE 5.1 *Frequency of sex chromosomal anomalies*

Anomaly	Rate per 1000 births
Boys	
XYY (extra Y syndrome)	1.0
XXY (Kleinfelter's syndrome)	1.0
Girls	
XXX (triple X syndrome)	1.0
Both sexes, miscellaneous other	0.5

SOURCE: Peckham, Ross and Farmer, 1982

with an overall incidence rate of 1.5 per 1000 births, though the rate rises rapidly in older mothers. Although many Down's syndrome babies survive, they do have an above-average infant mortality. Almost all babies born with other autosomal anomalies die in infancy.

MEASURING INFANT DEATHS

Many embryos with a genetic disorder are lost during pregnancy. Others, like the normal majority of foetuses, survive in the womb to be born. But the first year of life is still a comparatively vulnerable period, as our earlier examination of infant mortality showed. And the risks are often different for male and female babies. We shall therefore begin our detailed look at women's health at different ages by studying the major health risks for females – and how far they are different from male health risks – in the first year of life.

There are a number of different measurements which cover aspects of death to babies under one year of age.

Stillbirths – defined as late foetal deaths after 28 weeks gestation, and *perinatal deaths* – stillbirths and deaths in the first week of life – are measured as the rate per 1000 live and still births.
Neonatal deaths – deaths in the first 28 days of life – and
postneonatal deaths – the rest of the period to the child's first birthday – are measured in rates per 1000 live births.
The Infant Mortality Rate covers all deaths under one year of age, i.e. neonatal plus post-neonatal, and it is also measured per 1000 live births.

SEX DIFFERENCES IN INFANTS' RISK OF DEATH

Infant mortality has declined very rapidly in England and Wales, in common with most other developed countries, during the course of the century. Today, one in a hundred babies dies before its first birthday, compared with over ten per cent in 1910–12 (OPCS, 1986). In the developing world, sadly, that figure of ten per cent – or even more – is still not uncommon. High though that figure is, it does represent some progress: until forty or fifty years ago, probably around one in five children did not survive their first year in the less-developed countries.

The extra resilience of female babies is apparent in the stillbirth and perinatal death rates for England and Wales in 1983. The stillbirth rate was 5.4 per 1000 births for females, compared with 6.0 for males, and the perinatal rate was 9.6 per 1000 female births, compared with 11.1 for males.

The sex difference in death rates is even more marked in the death rates of twins (Table 5.2). All same-sex twins (formed from a single egg) are more likely to die after a live birth than non-identical twins, but the rates are considerably lower for female than for male pairs.

TABLE 5.2 *Twin births in England and Wales, 1982: mortality rates per 1000 total births*

	Two males	One male one female	Two females
Stillbirths	22.6	13.6	22.7
Perinatal deaths	59.4	28.4	44.7
Neonatal deaths	42.9	18.1	26.7
Postneonatal deaths	12.2	8.9	10.5
Infant deaths	55.1	27.0	37.3

SOURCE: OPCS, 1986

For both boys and girls, the early days and weeks of life are those in which they are at greatest risk. After the first two months of life the number of deaths decreases quite sharply (Table 5.3). But the differential between the two sexes increases again towards the end of the first year.

TABLE 5.3 *Infant deaths, by sex and months of age: England and Wales 1984*

	Age (months)			
	1–2	*3–5*	*6–8*	*9–11*
Males	588	468	204	135
Females	461	374	168	95
ratio m/f	1.28	1.25	1.21	1.42

SOURCE: POCS, 1986a

CAUSES OF INFANT DEATHS

The causes of death to infants are not generally very different by sex.
The most frequent causes of death for infants of both sexes are risks
related to *complications of pregnancy, childbirth*, and so on, and
congenital abnormalities (a death rate of around 2.5 per 1000 births)
which together make up about a quarter of infant deaths.

In almost a further quarter of all infant deaths the cause is not
clearly identified, and the deaths are grouped under the residual
group of *signs, symptoms and ill-defined conditions*. Cot deaths are
about a fifth more common among boys than girls, though between
1983 and 1984 the rate for girls was rising while that for boys
declined. Cot deaths are the single most common cause of infant
death after the first month of life. When autopsies are carried out on
the victims, about a third are found to have suffered from some
illness, including sudden infectious disease, and some of the
remainder have previously undiagnosed congenital abnormalities. 'A
few have ineffectual parents, but much more commonly they are
normal caring parents . . .' (Peckham, Ross and Farmer 1982a) and
the cause of many of these tragedies remains unclear.

Deaths of infants are not spread evenly among all socio-economic
groups: the differences between social classes are, in fact, dramatic.
While overall infant mortality in 1983 in England and Wales was 9.4
per 1000 legitimate live births, the rate for social class I was only 6.2
while that of social class V was 12.8. Deaths from *respiratory*
infections were more than twice as common in social class V than in
class I and cot deaths three times as common.

Congenital abnormalities

Many foetuses with *congenital abnormalities* are lost in pregnancy – estimates suggest that about 40 per cent of all spontaneous
abortions involve the loss of faulty embryos. However, it is also
estimated that up to five per cent of live births show some genetic or
developmental anomaly, and major malformations are involved in
two per cent of live births (Peckham, Ross and Farmer, 1982a). The
most common types of major malformation found at birth in Britain
are given in Table 5.4.

Girls in England and Wales seem to be more prone to death from
anencephalus (malformation of the skull with absence of a brain) and
to deaths from other abnormalities.

TABLE 5.4   *Approximate frequency and sex ratio of the more common major congenital abnormalities in Britain*

Malformations	Frequency per 1000 births	Male: female ratio
Spina bifida cystica	2.5	0.6
Anencephaly	2.0	0.3
Congenital heart defects	6.0	1.0
Pyloric stenosis	3.0	4.0
Cleft lip (with or without cleft palate)	1.0	1.8
Congenital dislocation of the hip (late diagnosis)	1.0	0.14

SOURCE: Peckham, Ross and Farmer, 1982

Spina bifida cystica combines a defect of the spinal wall and the protrusion of the spinal cord. It is often associated with hydrocephalus (cerebro-spinal fluid in the skull), and is found almost twice as often in girls as boys. Pyloric stenosis is a narrowing or blockage of the lower opening of the stomach.

Neural tube defects, and particularly malformations of the brain and spinal cord, vary enormously in their distribution internationally as well as within Britain. Even within this comparatively small island there are large regional variations in the rates for some of these abnormalities. The incidence of anencephaly ranges from 1.5 per 1000 live births in south-east England to three per 1000 in Wales and Scotland. Ireland has still higher rates, of four per 1000 in Ulster, and six in the Republic. Deaths from neural tube defects are 20 times as high in Ulster as in Japan or Portugal. This is an indication that there may be some environmental factor contributing to many of these malformations. They also seem to involve a genetic factor – where a couple have a spina bifida baby, for example, there is a 5–8 per cent chance that any further child they have will have a major malformation of the central nervous system. But they also vary by social class, being more common in the lower socio-economic groups. The diet of the mother during pregnancy is also suspected as having an influence.

Perinatal deaths

Congenital abnormalities are more likely to cause the death of male babies during the first week of life. This is a reversal of the situation in spontaneous abortion, when more females are likely to be lost from these causes.

During the first week, boys are, in addition, more likely to die from a group of causes such as respiratory distress syndrome. On average, it appears that male babies are, at a given gestational age, less mature and have less developed lungs, and this may explain their susceptibility to respiratory problems, both in the first week and later.

Low birthweight is a factor underlying many of the stillbirths and perinatal deaths. The term low birthweight covers babies who are small for their gestational age – because they have not developed fully, or are multiple births, or have a congenital defect – and infants born prematurely. Although it is possible that there are genetic differences between different races in the size of a full-term infant (WHO, 1980), social and economic factors seem to be much more important in low birthweight babies.

One of these factors is smoking. Cigarette smoking in pregnancy affects the birthweight at a given gestational age (Peckham, Ross and Farmer, 1982) as well as increasing the risk of perinatal mortality by between four and 40 per cent (de Scrill et. al., 1986). Very young mothers also tend to have low birthweight babies, as do mothers with a poor or inadequate diet.

In England and Wales in 1983, babies weighing less than 2500 gm at delivery accounted for almost two-thirds of all stillbirths and perinatal deaths (OPCS, 1986). There were no real differences by sex in the proportions of low birthweight babies amongs stillbirths or perinatal deaths.

Post-neonatal deaths

Deaths at the older stages of infancy are primarily from *respiratory diseases* – males aged 9–11 months were more than twice as likely to succumb to these as were females – congenital anomalies and sudden deaths including cot deaths. Males of six months or over were also much more likely to die from *injury or accidental poisoning*. It is rather surprising that there should be a sex bias in this last group of deaths. Boys and young men have higher rates of accident and injury, and in earlier chapters it was pointed out that boys may be encouraged to behave in a more adventurous fashion, and to be 'tougher', than girls. However, it is difficult to imagine such influences operating strongly on infants. It is generally considered, though, that boys begin to crawl and walk a little earlier than girls, which may put them at risk at an earlier stage.

SEX DIFFERENTIALS IN INFANT MORTALITY IN DEVELOPING COUNTRIES

Because of the poor quality of birth and death registration in many developing countries, accurate statistics on infant mortality are not easy to get. But one study (Heligman, 1983) of 22 countries for which there were a total of 36 life tables compiled at different times, found that the ratio of male to female infant deaths averaged 1.18. There were only two countries in which the ratio of male deaths did not exceed the female ones: those were India and Iran which, during the early 1970s, had ratios of 0.97 and 0.91, respectively.

These latter ratios do not come as a surprise, although they are an exception to the general pattern around the world. The earlier chapters have already demonstrated that the Indian subcontinent has long been known to have exceptionally high levels of female mortality, and that statistics in other countries in the past also showed more males than females surviving.

It is possible to look in more detail at this female disadvantage in infant death rates in a part of another country of the Indian subcontinent. There is a rural area of Bangladesh, covering 228 villages situated largely in Matlab county, where the International Centre for Diarrhoeal Disease Control operates a comprehensive registration system of births, marriages and deaths, and also routinely collects other demographic and health information.

During part of the period described in Table 5.5, Matlab – in common with much of Bangladesh – suffered a severe famine, in 1974–75. Even in normal times, however, the country is a desperately poor and underdeveloped one. If we look first at a normal year, 1977, Matlab had an infant mortality rate of 113.3 for males and 114.4 for females. However, when the deaths are divided into neonatal and post-neonatal, it can be seen that the excess female deaths occur only after the first month.

The *lower female neonatal mortality rates* suggest that the standard biological risk of excess male deaths during the first 28 days exists in Bangladesh as in other countries. The *higher death rate of girl infants after the first month* has been attributed to strong son-preference

TABLE 5.5   *Infant mortality rates, by sex, in Matlab, Bangladesh, 1974–77*

	1974	1975	1976	1977
Infant mortality rate:				
male	142.5	165.1	113.6	113.3
female	132.9	184.1	110.3	114.2
ratio m/f	1.07	0.90	1.03	0.99
Neonatal mortality rate:				
male	87.9	81.6	72.0	73.1
female	67.8	78.12	58.1	69.4
ratio m/ı	1.30	1.04	1.24	1.05
Postneonatal mortality rate:				
male	54.6	98.4	33.3	40.2
female	65.1	126.3	42.1	44.8
ratio m/f	0.84	0.78	0.79	0.90

SOURCE: D'Souza and Chen, 1980

among Bangladeshis, which means that girls get a lower level of parental care, and may not be fed so frequently or treated so promptly if they become ill.

During the famine period, girls aged 1–11 months fared much worse than usual, and worse than male babies did. In a normal year like 1977, the excess mortality among girls was around 11 per cent; it reached 28 per cent in 1975. This suggests that at a time of severe deprivation, the crisis fell disproportionately on female babies. Evidence from other countries tends to support this finding: where girls have a low value, they have the lowest priority in a crisis (Kane, 1988).

There do not seem to be any particular sex differences in the *causes* of infant death in Bangladesh. Among the causes which were reasonably well identified in Matlab, neonatal tetanus accounted for a quarter of all deaths in infancy, while deaths from measles, and from respiratory and diarrhoeal diseases were also common. The usual greater male vulnerability to infections in infancy, which was discussed earlier, is not visible here: female death rates from measles and respiratory diseases are higher. Poorer care and nutrition of girl babies in countries like Bangladesh can reverse their biological or genetic advantage and leave them open to infections and subsequent death.

The kind of pattern of infant deaths given here for Matlab, in which males show excess deaths only in the first month of life and females have the higher overall infant mortality rate, has occurred in other countries – including some Western ones – in the past.

We have seen that there was excess female child and adult mortality in Germany at various periods between the sixteenth and nineteenth centuries. In England, in the mid and late nineteenth century, the death rate of young girls was abnormally high. In these situations, too, the excess female deaths have been attributed to the social and economic disadvantages of women and girls, especially at the lower social levels, and to deliberate or unconscious neglect of girl babies by parents.

DEATHS DURING CHILDHOOD

After the first year of life, the risk of death begins to fall. While about one in every hundred infants die, only about four in every 10 000 children aged 1–4 in low mortality countries do so. This age group in turn has twice the risk of death of children aged 5–14. Probably as a reflection of these changing levels of risk, child deaths are usually divided into those two age-groups.

In England and Wales in 1984, there were 42.4 deaths among every 100 000 children aged 1–4, compared to 21.9 deaths for every 100 000 children in the older ages 5–14. The rates for girls were lower than for boys, and the difference increased with increasing age. Mortality rates at ages 1–4 were 37 per 100 000 for girls and 47 for boys; at ages 5–14 they were 18 per 100 000 for girls and 26 for boys.

CAUSES OF DEATH

The most common cause of death in England and Wales, among children aged 1–4, for both sexes, is still some *congenital anomaly*. Such abnormalities produced,in 1984 a mortality rate of 9.3 per 100 000 population in this age group; in other words, congenital anomalies accounted for almost a quarter of all deaths. Babies who are born with severe defects may increasingly, as the result of modern medical techniques, survive infancy – but not the childhood years.

The second most common cause is death due to *accidents*, with a rate of 8.6 per 100 000 population aged 1–4. Third among the

common causes of death are deaths from *cancers*, which produce
mortality of six per 100 000 population in this age group. Leukaemias
are the major contributor to the cancer deaths, and most frequent
among them is acute lymphatic leukaemia.

Among children in England and Wales aged 5–14 in 1984, *accidents*
rise to first place as a cause of death (8.6 per 100 000) followed by
cancers (4.4 per 100 000) – again, largely leukaemias – and *congenital anomalies* fall to third place, with a rate of 2.0 per 100 000.

Accidents and violence

Overall, among all children under 15 years, *accidents and violence*
– which are grouped together in the statistics – are the most common
cause of death. Two studies of child deaths in England and Wales
between 1968 and 1974 showed that more than half of the deaths
were due to transport accidents (Table 5.6).

The biggest group of those transport accidents was where a child
was hit by a car: this type of accident was relatively most common
among children aged 5–9, where it accounted for almost half of all
accidental deaths. Figures for 1978 show that road accidents among
children were much more common for boys than for girls.

It would seem that little boys are able to go about, either on foot or
on a bicycle, more freely and with less supervision than can little girls,
judging by the disparities in the numbers who die or are admitted to
hospital. This conclusion is borne out by the detailed study of child

TABLE 5.6 *Mortality and morbidity from road
accidents in England and Wales, 1978: rates per million population.*

Age	Death rates pedestrian	pedal cyclists	Hospital admissions all road accidents (rates)
Males			
0–4	41	3	935
5–14	54	18	1977
Females			
0–4	26	0	494
5–14	28	4	1033

SOURCE: Farmer, Nixon and Connolly, 1982

accidents leading to death or hospital treatment between 1968 and 1974 (MacFarlane, 1979) which showed that, even when transport accidents and homicide are excluded, smaller percentages of accidents to boys than girls took place inside the home. Boys who died outside the home were more often on farms, or in mines, quarries and industrial premises. The percentage of *accidental deaths in the home* among boys was 66.4 for those aged 1–4, and 22.5 for those aged 5–9. For girls the percentages were 76.3 and 53.5.

In 1984, in England and Wales, there were 81 deaths from accidents in the home among boys aged 1–4, and 49 among those aged 5–14. The comparable figures for girls were 49 and 25. Fire and flames are the most common domestic accidental cause of death in both age groups (with 45 boys and 30 girls dying), followed by suffocation (25 and 10), falls (15 and 5), and drowning (13 and 3). Boys also have a larger number of deaths from varied residual classification which is grouped together as 'other accidents': 11 deaths, compared with six (OPCS, 1986b). It seems that inside as well as outside the home boys are less likely to be generally supervised.

Although the numbers of deaths are quite small, they represent only the tip of the iceberg of accidental injury: fractures and head injuries result in about 7000 hospital admissions a year for the under-fives and burns result in a further 1000 admissions in the same age group.

Leukaemia

Caused by a failure of the body's controls on the proliferation of the white corpuscles in the blood, leukaemias may be either chronic or acute, and are described according to the type of corpuscles chiefly present. Around 28 per cent of all deaths from acute lymphatic leukaemia are to children under the age of ten. There are 1.7 male deaths from acute lymphatic leukaemia for every one female death (Berry, 1982). It is suspected that there may be some genetic predisposition to leukaemia and if this is so it could explain the large excess of male deaths in acute lymphatic leukaemia.

ILLNESS IN INFANCY AND CHILDHOOD

While deaths and death rates among those under the age of 15 are generally separated out into deaths occurring in infancy; deaths at ages 1–4; and deaths at ages 5–14, the information about childhood illness is grouped differently. It covers children aged 0–4 and 5–14, and thus means that infant illness, and early childhood illness, have to be examined together.

HOSPITAL EPISODES

As we saw in Chapter 3, children aged 0–4 have rather high rates of hospitalisation; older children have the lowest rates of any group in the population. Rates of hospital discharges (including those whose discharge is through death) for England in 1984 show that at all ages during childhood, males predominate (Table 5.7). They have higher discharge rates, and form a bigger proportion of the average number of beds used daily. However, their stay in hospital for a particular episode is shorter up to the age of ten, perhaps because more young male than female illnesses end in death.

TABLE 5.7 *Hospital discharges (including deaths) at ages 0–14, by sex: England 1984*

Category	0–4	5–9	10–14
Number in sample			
male	25 253	12 092	10 127
female	16 905	7 597	7 665
Discharge rates per 1000 population			
male	1 667.6	856.1	592.7
female	1 173.6	568.4	473.3
ratio m/f	1.42	1.51	1.25
Average number of beds used daily per million population			
male	2 158	784	1 010
female	1 688	543	588
ratio m/f	1.28	1.44	1.72
Mean duration of stay			
male	4.7	3.4	6.2
female	5.3	3.5	4.5

SOURCE: DHSS, 1986

There are some causes of illness or death which lead to higher discharge rates among children (especially very young children) than among the population as a whole. They are, in other words, the causes of illness or death which apply particularly to children. Rates given in brackets are ones where the rates for children do not exceed the overall rates; they are included for comparison. The more important groups by diagnosis are given below: all of them show *higher rates for males* than for female children.

TABLE 5.8 *Hospital discharge rates per 10 000 children, by age and sex, for major diagnostic groups in which the age-specific rate exceeds the rate at all ages: England 1984*

	Male		Female	
Diagnostic group	0–4	5–14	0–4	5–14
Infectious and parasitic	89.7	(15.3)	71.6	(11.1)
Respiratory system	351.6	125.4	217.6	114.4
D. of other parts of digestive system	128.0	(47.0)	(71.6)	(31.7)
Congenital anomalies	131.1	49.8	84.1	19.3
Perinatal	207.6	(0.4)	182.8	(0.0)
Signs, symptoms and ill-defined conditions	271.5	(95.1)	208.2	(83.1)
Injuries and poisoning	183.3	157.1	139.2	(84.4)

Note: bracketed rates do not exceed the rates at all ages and are given for comparison.
SOURCE: DHSS, 1986

Under the heading of *infectious and parasitic diseases*, it is in-testinal infections which account for the majority of the hospitalised illnesses experienced by young boys, as well as for just under half of those experienced by girls.

In the category of *respiratory diseases*, boys aged 0–4 have twice the rate of hospitalisation for bronchitis, asthma and emphysema, and also have higher rates for pneumonia. However, girls are somewhat more likely to have a hospital episode involving chronic diseases of the tonsils or adenoids.

The category *diseases of other parts of the digestive system* includes appendicitis and hernia. While discharge rates for appendicitis peak for both sexes in the age group 5–14, boys of that age have a rate of 23.2 per 10 000 while that for girls of the same age is 17.7. In the 0–4 age group, hernias among boys are more than four times as common a cause of a hospital episode as are hernias in girls.

We have already seen that boys are more likely to die in infancy, and their greater vulnerability helps to account for the higher rates of discharge under the headings of *congenital anomalies*, and of *conditions originating in the perinatal period*. But quite a large contribution to the male excess of hospital discharges from congenital anomalies at ages 0–4 and 5–14 comes from those treated for an undescended testicle (21.2 and 24.4 per 10 000 respectively). Girls show marginally higher rates of spina bifida and hydrocephalus.

A major contribution to discharges under the heading of *conditions originating in the perinatal period* is hypoxia, birth asphyxia and other respiratory conditions; both aged 0–4 have a discharge rate of 53.2 compared with 42.4 for girls.

Children, especially very small children who are unable to speak or express themselves clearly, are not always easy to diagnose, and this explains the high rates of child hospitalisation under the category of *signs, symptoms and ill-defined conditions*. Within that general category, girls are slightly more likely to be classified as having abdominal pain.

We have also seen that boys have higher death rates than girls from accidents. Boys aged 0–4 and 5–14 are more likely to have a hospital episode as the result of *injury or poison*; when the figures are examined in more detail, they show boys having higher rates for each of the sub-categories under those headings: fractures, internal injuries, open wounds and burns.

Other conditions

There are a few other diagnositic categories where children show higher rates of hospitalisation than do the rest of the population, although their contribution to the overall rates of hospital discharges is small.

Boys aged 0–4 and 5–9 (but not girls) have higher rates for disorders of the *blood*, and of the *skin*. Boys alone, of course, present themselves with diseases of the *male genital organs* and, in the age group 0–4, have a rate of complaint under this heading which is well above that of the male population as a whole: closer examination, however, shows that most of the hospital episodes are not for illness but for circumcision.

Girls have higher hospital discharge rates for one diagnostic group only, that of disorders of the *eye*, and most of the excess is due to strabismus (squint). Whether there really is a greater incidence of squinting among girls, or whether corrective action is seen to be more necessary when it is to improve the appearance of a girl, is not clear.

Thus a more comprehensive study of hospital episodes among children reinforces the view, suggested in the earlier chapters, that girls are less likely to suffer a serious episode of illness, leading to a stay in hospital, than are boys.

ILLNESS AS SEEN BY THE GENERAL PRACTITIONER

We can now turn to episodes of illness among children as seen by the general practitioner, and concentrate, again, on those illnesses where children have a higher rate than does the population as a whole (Table 5.9).

TABLE 5.9 *Rates of episode of GP attention per 1000 at risk, by age and sex, for those major diagnostic groups in which the age-specific rate at ages 0–14 exceeds that of the population: England and Wales 1981–2*

	Male		Female	
Diagnostic group	0–4	5–14	0–4	5–14
Infectious and parasitic	443.9	196.5	450.5	218.5
Nervous system	596.2	205.5	533.5	238.5
Respiratory	1261.0	537.1	1111.4	538.3
Digestive system	115.2	(33.7)	104.0	(34.4)
Genito-urinary	51.3	(24.2)	(40.3)	(43.2)
Skin, etc.	265.2	(122.3)	248.1	(147.2)
Congenital anomalies	21.4	6.3	14.0	3.0
Perinatal	5.5	(0.1)	2.8	(0.0)
Signs, symptoms and ill-defined	404.1	(175.0)	374.2	(188.1)
Accidents, poisoning, etc.	(137.3)	152.4	(109.7)	120.2

SOURCE: RCGP, 1986

It is apparent that the broad diagnostic headings for groups of illnesses which put a child into contact with a GP are very similar to those which result in hospitalisation. However, it is also clear that, while the rates of GP episode are generally higher for boys than for girls, the difference is not so great as it is for hospital episodes. In addition, there are at least two instances where the difference in rate favours boys. In contrast to the pattern seen in hospitals, girls throughout childhood have more frequent contact with a GP for *infectious and parasitic diseases*, and those aged 5–14 also show higher rates for diseases of the *nervous system*.

The picture becomes somewhat easier to understand when the illnesses which children suffer are examined in more detail. Broad diagnostic groupings cover quite a range of specific conditions; it is these specific conditions which are needed to compare or contrast hospital and GP episodes, or the illnesses suffered by each sex.

The *infectious and parasitic* diseases seen by GPs to which children are particularly prone are – as you would expect – *intestinal* infections, unspecified viral infections, whooping cough, chickenpox, polio, measles, rubella (German measles), mumps, and thrush. There are no very marked sex differences in the rates for these, although there is generally a slight preponderance of girls. Taken in conjunction with the figures for hospital episodes, this suggests that boys are more likely to end up in hospital, where girls are treated at home.

Diseases of the nervous system which result in children's disproportionate use of a GP include conjunctivitis, ear inflammations and strabismus. There are no marked sex differences in these rates.

Respiratory diseases include upper respiratory tract infections, tonsillitis, laryngitis, bronchitis, catarrh, hay fever and asthma. Boys have the higher rates for each of these conditions, with the exception of upper respiratory tract infections where girls aged 5–14 predominate.

Digestive diseases include tooth and mouth problems, irritable bowel syndrome, constipation and hernia. The last in the list, hernia, is overwhelmingly a complaint of boys aged 0–4.

Circumcision, though seldom required for medical reasons, figures largely among GP episodes classed under diseases of the *genito-urinary system*, along with balanitis (inflammation around the foreskin).

The main *skin* complaints are impetigo, nappy rash, dermatitis or eczema, nettle rash and (among girls aged 5–14) acne. Generally, boys show higher rates of skin diseases at the younger ages with the balance evening out in the 5–14 age group.

Undescended testicles produce the major contribution to sex differences in *congenital abnormalities* for which a GP is condulted.

Signs, symptoms and ill-defined conditions include convulsions, speech disturbances, heart murmurs, enlarged lymph nodes, anorexia or other feeding problems, failure to thrive, and bedwetting, but the main causes of the large number of children's complaints which come under this category are coughs, stomach pains and unexplained fevers and rashes. Girls have higher rates of stomach pain, and boys of bedwetting, but the other conditions show no particular pattern of sex differences.

Although the 5–14 age group does have a high level of accidents, poisoning and injuries, the conditions for which the GP treats a child tend to be the less serious ones. They involve sprains, bruises, cuts and head injuries or concussion, burns and scalds. Male children are more likely to require treatment for each of these conditions.

Overall, the rates for episodes of illness seen by a GP confirm the picture of greater male vulnerability, especially at the youngest ages. They show that there is less imbalance in the amount of illness between the sexes than the figures for deaths or hospitalisation imply.

ILLNESS IN THE COMMUNITY

The Australian Health Survey of 1983 (ABS, 1986 and ABS, 1986a) gives us a further perspective on the amount of illness among children, by sex. Where it was claimed that a person had experienced an illness in the two weeks before the interview, the respondents were asked whether or not they had done anything about it. In the case of children, their parents had usually taken some action (Table 5.10).

Boys under the age of five who experienced some illness were more likely to be taken to a doctor, or to another health professional, and/or given some medication. However, the survey suggests that there may be more illness among girls aged 0–5 than figures for consultations with health professionals indicate. In other words, the illnesses of boys seem to be taken more seriously, and considered to be more in need of expert attention, than are those of girls.

TABLE 5.10 *Types of health-related action taken for children experiencing one or more illness conditions in the two weeks prior to interview, by sex: Australia, 1983*

| | Numbers in thousands | | | |
| Types of action | males | | females | |
	0–4	5–14	0–4	5–14
Episode in hospital	3.4*	5.4*	3.3*	3.1*
Doctor consultation	125.9	140.0	113.5	143.8
Dental consultation	3.4*	51.1	2.1*	66.5
Consultation with another health professional	55.8	55.3	53.9	56.9
Medication taken	305.6	491.3	282.5	506.4
Day away from school		157.1		160.3
Day of reduced activities(a)	33.6	146.3	37.6	148.0

*sample size small; the estimated number is unreliable.
(a) asked only for those aged 2 and over.

SOURCE: ABS, 1986

SUMMARY AND CONCLUSIONS

What can we conclude about sex differences in health impairment among children? The higher male than female death rates in infancy appear to be caused by a combination of genetic, often sex-based, differences, and by social and economic factors which – in some countries – can considerably reduce, and even occasionally eliminate, the female advantage.

It seems that among the 0–5 age group, boys are given more medication, taken to doctors or other health professionals more often, and are more likely to have an episode in hospital. As they also have higher death rates than girls, much of their excess use of health-care services obviously results from their greater vulnerability. But it is also just possible that some of this extra care results from discriminatory anxiety about the health of a male child. The general belief that boys are more vulnerable may in itself produce more attention to the health of a boy. There are a few slight indications in the statistics that such discrimination may be a factor.

The Australian health survey (ABS, 1986a) asked parents who reported that they had not taken any action over the illness a child experienced during the two weeks before interview, why they had not done so. Where the child aged 0–5 was a boy, 58 per cent said the illness was not serious enough to warrant action; where the child was a girl, the percentage was 68. The GP survey in England and Wales showed more male than female children being taken to a doctor with unexplained minor conditions.

Another possible indication that the illnesses of young boys receive greater attention is that they seem to be more likely to be taken into hospital because of family circumstances or with conditions which are never clearly diagnosed. The International Classification of Diseases has a supplementary category covering *other reasons for contact with health services*. One of the codes under this heading is for *housing, household and economic circumstances*. The Hospital In-patient Inquiry for England shows the discharge rates under this heading as being 4.8 per 10 000 for boys aged 0–5, and 3.3 for girls. As we have already seen, the survey also suggested a greater likelihood that a boy would be hospitalised with *signs, symptoms and ill-defined conditions*.

Thus there do seem to be grounds for concluding that the community holds rather contradictory views about the care of male children. On the one hand, boys are allowed – even encouraged – to roam outside the home, and to behave in ways which lead to much higher risk of *accidents and injury* than girls have. On the other, their health problems seem to result in a more prompt use of professionals, and a greater referral to hospitals. Some of these male health problems, it is true, stem from the greater male vulnerability in childhood – to *infections and respiratory diseases* in particular. Some of the excess use of services by male children also results from purely *biological factors*, such as undescended testicles, inflammations of the foreskin, hernias and circumcision. But some of the remainder is difficult to explain other than by assuming differential care for male and female children.

6 Female Health in Early Adulthood

This chapter, and the next, draw largely on British and Australian statistics to illustrate the health status of adult females in the more developed countries. It is difficult to compare adult health in the industrialised world with that of men and women in the developing countries, for the simple reason that the necessary statistics in those countries are either non-existent, or so limited that one cannot make the type of detailed breakdown which is required here. The broad picture of adult mortality in the third world – virtually the only information available from which to draw inferences about health status – and glimpses of the use men and women make of medical services, has already been given in the first half of the book. It is just not possible to make the more specific comparisons which would be illuminating here.

FERTILITY

The biggest change in health and mortality for women of the industrialised world in the age group 15–44 has come, over the past fifty years or so, from changes in fertility. In Australia during the 1920s, for example, deaths due to childbirth were still among the five main causes of death of women aged 25–44 (Young and Ruzicka, 1982). Today, in Australia as in England, deaths due to childbirth are less than one in 10 000 confinements. Over the same period, family size for the various generations of women has fallen from almost five children to around two. Compare these figures with those from the Bangladesh surveys described in the second chapter and you will get an idea of how dramatic the change has been.

   The *reduction in maternal deaths* is due partly to improved medical care both antenatal and post-natal, use of antibiotics, and so on. However, it has also been substantially reduced through a combination of postponing marriage and childbearing to a more mature age, and reductions in the number of children couples have, which involves steep reductions in fertility at the later ages. Reduced fertility, in turn, owes much to increasingly available and effective contraceptives and more recently sterilisation. Since the 1960s, there has also been increased provision of legal abortion in industrialised countries.

It is true that women across Europe, as well as in North America and Australia, started to have fewer children from as early as the last decades of the 19th century. In order to have smaller families, they seem to have had to rely heavily on illegal – and often dangerous – abortions (Hicks, 1978), or on giving up sex altogether once they had the number of children they wanted (Ruzicka and Caldwell, 1977). The more widespread availability of contraception, and more convenient contraceptives, helped to speed up the pace of change. The introduction of the contraceptive Pill and the IUD, in particular, meant that women no longer had to rely on a partner for pregnancy prevention, but could control their own fertility. They made it easier for women to have only those children they wanted, and the choices they offered perhaps also affected women's views about how many children they did want.

Since the 1960s there has been an intensification of change in sexual attitudes and behaviour in Britain, as in many industrialised countries. The age at which women first have sexual intercourse has fallen, and there have been rises in the numbers experiencing premarital sexual intercourse, and in living with a man outside marriage.

In one survey carried out in England in 1964, 16 per cent of a sample of those aged 15–19 said they had sexual intercourse (Schofield, 1965). By 1974/5, another survey in England and Wales found that 42 per cent of those single girls aged 16–19 admitted to having had intercourse (Dunnell, 1979). More recently, a survey of family planning in Scotland found that the proportion of single girls aged 15–19 who had experienced sexual intercourse had risen from about 7 per cent in 1964 to over 20 per cent in 1981 (Bone, 1986).

Among women in Britain who married between 1956 and 1960, just over a third had premarital sex with their future husband; among women marrying between 1971 and 1975, the proportion was three quarters (Dunnell, 1979). The General Household Survey found that in Britain in 1979, about a fifth of marriages between bachelors and spinsters involved couples who had previously cohabited: even where the bride was under 20 the proportion was 9 per cent (Haskey and Coleman, 1986).

Age at marriage

One reason for the increasing proportions of young women having premarital sex or living with a man is that the age at marriage has been rising, for both males and females. The median age at marriage for men in England and Wales which had been 24.1 years in 1971, was 26.7 years in 1985. For women, the comparable figures are 22.0 and 24.3 years.

Postponement of childbearing

Partly because of this postponement of marriage, there has also been a postponement of childbearing. In England and Wales in 1977, there were 29.4 births for every 1000 women aged under 20, 103.7 for those aged 20–24, and 117.5 in the age group 25–29. By 1985, the comparable numbers of live births for every 1000 women were 29.5, 94.5 and 127.6; in other words the peak period for childbearing was increasingly at ages 25–29. With smaller families also becoming the norm, the average age of mothers at childbirth (all births) is now 27 years (OPCS, 1986c).

Contraception

Reductions in the age of first intercourse, and delays in the age of marriage, increase the period in which a woman is at risk of conception outside marriage. The Scottish family planning survey (Bone, 1986) found that for women born before 1951, the median time between first sexual experience and marriage was 15 months, while it was over two years for women born between 1956 and 1960. There still too often remains a gap between beginning sexual intercourse and use of contraception. Even in the most recent cohort (those born in 1961–5), more than a quarter of those aged under 20 had their first pre-marital sex without protection.

On the other hand, whereas almost none of the women born prior to 1941 had used contraception *before* their first sexual experience, around 40 per cent of those born in 1956–60 had done so. To some extent, it is unfair to compare these recent cohorts with the women born before 1941, who would have become sexually active in the late 1950s, before the Pill became widely available and before family planning clinics and GPs were willing to see unmarried women. Increased use of contraception – whether from the time of first intercourse, or only after some months of sexual experience – has reduced the probability of young, single women becoming pregnant. At the time of the survey, only three percent of the single girls who had experienced intercourse in the previous twelve months were not protected by contraception on the last occasion.

This alteration in sexual behaviour, including the timing of marriage, pregnancy and use of contraception, has had its effects on various aspects of health: some of these are discussed later in the chapter. Most of the statistics discussed in this chapter split men and women into two groups – those aged 15–24, and those aged 25–44. When looking at the figures on use of health services by women, it is worth bearing in mind that the first, younger, group are largely those who are beginning their sexual lives, and use of contraception, while the older group are those having and completing their families.

DEATHS IN YOUNG ADULTHOOD

Death rates in young adulthood, between the ages of 15 and 24, are almost the lowest for any ten-year age group in most countries. They are bettered only by the rates for those aged 5–14. Death rates per 100 000 population in England and Wales in 1984 for men aged 15–19 and 20–24 respectively were 71 and 84, while for women they were even lower, at 29 and 31.

CAUSES OF DEATH

The pattern of deaths by cause for age group 15–24 is rather more complex than might be suggested by the patterns which we have examined for whole populations in the earlier chapters. While it is clear that the lesser vulnerability of young women than men to accidents and injuries is an important reason for the much lower female death rates in young adulthood, it is not the only one. Women have *lower death rates* than men from *all* the significant causes of death – including cancer.

Table 6.1 shows *accidental deaths, injuries and poisoning* as the overwhelming contributors to the death rates at this age, especially for men. The male death rate from this category is more than four times that of the women.

TABLE 6.1   *Major causes of death at ages 15–24, rates per 100 000 population, by sex: England 1984*

Cause of death	Male	Female
All causes	76.3	29.2
Infectious and parasitic	0.9	0.8
Neoplasms	7.7	5.1
Endocrine, nutritional and metabolic	1.1	1.0
Mental disorders	1.3	0.4
Nervous system	4.5	1.9
Circulatory	3.4	2.1
Respiratory	2.3	1.5
Digestive	0.8	0.6
Congenital anomalies	1.9	1.7
Injuries and poisoning	51.4	12.7

SOURCE: OPCS, 1986d

Accidents are the major single cause of death in the age group 15–24 in many countries, as we saw in Chapter 2. In 1985 in England and Wales, there were a total of 527 deaths for every million people aged 15–24, of which 234 – or almost half – were due to accidents (OPCS 1986c). In turn, almost three-fifths of these accidental deaths arose from motor accidents. Women were far less likely to be killed in motor accidents: the death rate was 303.9 for every million men aged 15–24, and 72.2 for women. A further fifth of deaths under the heading of accidents, injuries and poisoning were due to suicide. Suicide will be discussed a little further on, as the rates peak in the next age-groups.

One important contribution to the accident figures is the use of alcohol. A recent survey of adolescents in Britain reported that about a quarter of boys aged 13 report drinking alcohol at least weekly, and by age 17 the proportion had risen to more than half. However, a majority of girls aged 13 had drunk no alcohol in the week which was studied in detail, and at all ages the girls drank less (OPCS 1987). A slightly earlier survey of the drinking habits of women aged 18 or over (Breeze, 1985) found that most adult women drank little or nothing during the week prior to interview. The very few women who did drink heavily tended to be unmarried and under the age of 25, or married but without young children at home. Stress, rather than boredom or isolation, was the main reason given for heavy drinking.

The second most frequent cause of death at this age, though it makes up only a fraction of the mortality from external causes, is *cancer*. The leukaemias are the biggest factor in cancer deaths in this age group, with a rate of 18.7 for every million men and 11.2 for women. Acute lymphatic leukaemia is found more frequently among males than females, as we saw in the previous chapter. We also noted that there may be a genetic predisposition to the development of leukaemia, as it is associated with a number of specific chromosomal abnormalities (Berry, 1982).

DEATHS AGED 25–44

Death rates are also comparatively low for those aged 25–44 (Table 6.2), although they begin to increase over that age-span. Those for

TABLE 6.2   *Death rates at ages 25–44 per 100 000 population, by sex: England and Wales 1984*

Age	Male	Female	M/F ratio
25–29	82	42	1.95
30–34	93	57	1.63
35–39	128	86	1.49
40–44	213	143	1.49

SOURCE: OPCS, 1986d

men aged 25–29 are actually lower (82 per 100 000 population) than the rates for men aged 20–24, because there are fewer deaths due to accidents and injuries among this older group. Women preserve their advantage in each five-year age-group, although the extent of the advantage decreases somewhat after age 34.

Women's Health

CAUSES OF DEATH

Accidents and injuries, despite their less devastating incidence, are still the main cause of death for men aged 25–34, and the second most important cause for men aged 35–44 (Table 6.3).

TABLE 6.3   *Major causes of death at ages 25–44, rates per 100 000, by sex:*
England 1984

| | Male | | Female | |
Cause of death	25–34	35–44	25–34	35–44
All causes	85.9	162.3	48.5	110.0
Infectious and parasitic	0.9	1.5	1.0	1.0
Neoplasms	13.9	40.1	17.8	57.9
Endocrine, nutritional and metabolic	1.4	2.4	1.2	1.6
Mental disorders	2.1	1.9	0.9	0.6
Nervous system	3.9	4.6	3.2	4.2
Circulatory	10.8	54.0	5.5	17.5
Respiratory	2.7	4.9	2.1	3.6
Digestive	2.3	7.1	1.5	4.0
Congenital anomalies	1.9	1.5	1.1	1.1
Injuries and poisoning	44.7	42.3	12.3	15.8

SOURCE: OPCS, 1986d

For women aged 25–34, *cancer* is the major cause of death, with *accidents and injuries* coming second to cancer. Amongst women aged 35–44, although the mortality rate from *accidents and injuries* actually increases, they fall to third place in prominence, following both *cancer* and diseases of the *circulatory system*. The proportionate advantage in accident-related mortality which women have over men, though, declines with age: in other words, between ages 15 and 44, there is a steady decline in male death rates from accidents and injuries, while the decline for women is smaller and less consistent.

For both men and women in the age group 25–34, suicide is an important element in the category of injuries and poisoning; two in every five deaths under this heading are due to suicide. (Suicide, as we noted earlier, accounted for one in five of all deaths due to injury and poisoning among the age group 15–24.) There are about three times as many male suicides among men aged 25–34 as there are among women.

Although many people believe that suicide is primarily concentrated among young people, this is not in fact true. Suicide stands out as a major cause of death for young people, because their death rates from illnesses are so low, but the age-specific suicide rates are highest for *elderly* people. In other words, there are more suicides as a proportion of the elderly than there are among young people.

Over the past twenty years, however, the pattern of suicide in England and Wales has changed for men. Suicide rates among the elderly have fallen, while for younger men, especially those aged 25–44, those rates have risen. Among women, the pattern has been, and remains, one of lower rates than for men in general, and higher suicide rates at the older rather than younger ages. We shall discuss this further in Chapter 7.

There are differences between countries, and over time, as well as between men and women, in the ways suicide is carried out. In the 1950s in England and Wales, for example, domestic gas was the most common method of suicide for both sexes. The change to natural gas, which is much safer, has almost eliminated this method. By 1980, a third of male suicide deaths were due to hanging, strangulation or suffocation. Only a quarter of the deaths were due to poison, and a further nine per cent were due to firearms. Well over half of the female deaths, by contrast, resulted from poison; the majority of the remainder were due either to hanging, or to drowning (Bulusu and Alderson, 1984).

Deaths due to *cancer* rise very rapidly in both sexes in the age groups 25–44, especially in the decade 35–44. But whereas women below the age of 25 had lower rates of cancer than men, the pattern reverses itself here.

Among women aged 25–34, breast cancer and cancer of the cervix are already the leading causes of death, with leukaemia slipping to third place. The mortality rate from breast cancer rises to 21.1 per 100 000 in women aged 35–44, and from cancer of the cervix it increases to 6.5. Beginning sexual intercourse at an early age, early and frequent pregnancies, and number of sexual partners are all factors associated with cervical cancer. By contrast, breast cancer is more common in those who are childless or have their pregnancies comparatively late.

Men aged 35–44 have a mortality rate of 7.3 per 100 000 from lung cancer. Male death rates from most of the remaining cancers are higher – often, indeed, much higher – than those of women.

The main contributor to the deaths from *endocrine, nutritional and metabolic* disorders is diabetes mellitus; men are known to have slightly higher age-specific death rates from this disease and there is a genetic component to its causation (Florey, 1982).

The main cause of death from a disease of the *circulatory system* is, for both sexes, ischaemic heart disease. This produces death rates per 100 000 of 5.1 for men aged 25–34, and 39.2 for men aged 35–44. Women have much lower death rates from all diseases of the circulatory system, and while ischaemic heart disease is also the leading cause within that broader group, it makes a proportionately much smaller contribution to the lower female mortality rate.

Bronchitis, emphysema and asthma between them account for nearly half of the deaths due to *respiratory diseases*; their contributions are similar for men and women, although women in these age groups have lower death rates overall from these particular diseases.

Chronic liver disease, and cirrhosis of the liver, are major causes of death under the heading of diseases of the *digestive organs*. At ages 25–34, they make up about one third of male deaths in that category; by ages 35–44 they account for half of both the male and female deaths from diseases of the digestive system.

HOSPITAL EPISODES

Partly – but not entirely – because of their low death rates, young adults are, apart from children aged 5–9, the least likely group in the population to spend time in hospital. Hospital discharge rates for England in 1984 show low hospital-use by both sexes (DHSS, 1986). These discharge rates, it will be recalled, include deaths as well as all other outcomes of a hospital episode. They also show that there are more male than female hospital episodes for the age groups 15–19 and 20–24 (Table 6.4). Nevertheless, women have a slightly lower mean duration of stay in hospital in both age-groups.

Among those aged 25–44 (Table 6.5), discharge rates for women are rather stable, at 95–99 per 1000, and there is no pronounced age trend. Men's discharge rates, on the other hand, are virtually consistent at around 53–54 per 1000 between ages 25 and 40; at ages

TABLE 6.4   *Hospital episodes among those aged 15–24: England 1984*

Category	Male		Female		M/F ratio	
	15–19	*20–24*	*15–19*	*20–24*	*15–19*	*20–24*
Discharge rates per 10 000 population	558.0	582.3	721.3	879.9	0.77	0.66
Average number of beds used daily per million population	807	809	769	883	1.05	0.92
Mean duration of stay	5.3	5.1	3.9	3.7	1.36	1.38

SOURCE: DHSS, 1986

TABLE 6.5   *Hospital episodes among those aged 25–44: England 1984*

Category	Male				Female			
	25–29	*30–34*	*35–39*	*40–44*	*25–29*	*30–34*	*35–39*	*40–44*
Discharge rates per 10 000 population	539.1	533.4	537.1	619.4	976.1	993.5	946.6	977.3
M/F ratios	0.55	0.54	0.57	0.63				
Average no. of beds used daily per million pop.	787	843	1147	1129	1045	1202	1271	1654
M/F ratios	0.75	0.70	0.90	0.68				
Mean duration of stay	5.3	5.8	7.8	6.7	3.9	4.4	4.9	6.2
M/F ratios	1.77	1.32	1.59	1.08				

SOURCE: DHSS, 1986

40–44 their sharp increase to 62 per 1000 reduces the female excess. Women take up a larger proportion of the beds used daily than men. However, women continue to have shorter hospital stays than men until ages 40–44, when the difference becomes negligible.

Thus, from the age of 15 onwards, women are considerably more likely than men of the same age to spend some time in hospital, and, from about age 20, to take up a greater proportion of the average number of beds used daily. But, throughout the whole age-range from 15 to 44, they are in hospital for a shorter spell than men.

TABLE 6.6 *Discharges and deaths in hospital at ages 15–44, by sex and major diagnostic group, per 10 000 population: England 1984*

Diagnosis	Male	Female
All causes	548.5	852.0
Neoplasms	22.0	54.5
Respiratory	38.8	39.8
Digestive	58.6	51.2
Diseases of the female genital organs		169.1
Abortion: spontaneous		29.4
induced		45.3
Obstetric		28.9
Skin	17.4	15.6
Musculoskeletal	50.3	42.4
Signs, symptoms and ill-defined	79.5	129.8
Accidents, injuries	145.4	72.8
Sterilisation	3.2	43.8

SOURCE: DHSS, 1986

It is difficult to be sure of the reasons for the fluctuations in the pattern at different ages because, unfortunately, the report of the Hospital In-patient Enquiry does not provide a detailed age break-down of the causes of the hospital episodes, but groups the causes together for all those aged 15–44. We have, therefore, to be content with a general overview of the causes of hospital stay in young adulthood (Table 6.6).

Leaving aside, for the moment, the residual category of signs, symptoms and ill-defined conditions, it is apparent that – as was suggested in the earlier chapters – the *female reproductive system* is the predominant reason for women's high rates of hospitalisation in the fertile age groups. Even the neoplasms largely involve cancer of the breast, cervix and uterus.

Women are hospitalised for diseases of the female genital system, abortions and obstetric causes, and for sterilisation. Their rates of hospital discharge under these four headings total 287.6 per 10 000: in other words those four, specifically female, conditions account for one-third of their use of hospitals, and explain more than 95 percent of their excess hospitalisation.

By contrast, men have higher discharge rates for almost all of the diagnostic groups which are unconnected with reproduction, and especially for *accidents and injuries*. This probably explains their average longer durations of stay in hospital.

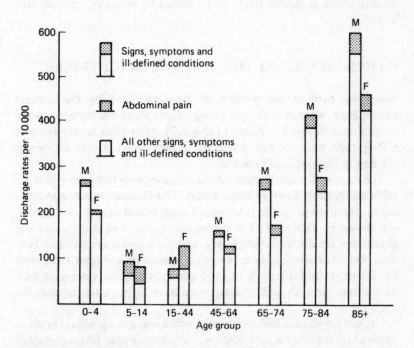

Figure 6.1 Hospital discharge rates per 10 000, by age and sex, for signs, symptoms amd ill-defined conditions: England, 1984.

SOURCE: DHSS, 1986.

Women do, however, have higher rates of hospitalisation for the residual group of *signs, symptoms and ill-defined conditions*. Among the symptoms reported by both sexes which are likely to result in examination in hospital, and which subsequently remain un-diagnosed, abdominal pain is common. At most ages, the differences between the sexes in hospital discharge rates for abdominal pain are small, as Figure 6.1 shows. However, between the ages of 15 and 44, women are almost three times as likely as men to be hospitalised under this heading.

It seems probable that here again it is concern about the female reproductive system which is being expressed. Both the woman and her doctor are likely to be alert to the possibility that abdominal pain may symptomise such conditions as, for example, pelvic inflamma-tory disease. There is some confirmation for this assumption in Figure 6.1. At all other ages more men that women have hospital episodes with undiagnosed conditions; women's excess in the repro-ductive years is indeed likely to be linked to issues of reproductive health.

ILLNESS AS SEEN BY THE GENERAL PRACTITIONER

When we turn to the pattern of illness as seen by the general practitioner, women in the age groups 15–44 also have higher episode rates almost across the board (Table 6.7). Men have higher rates of GP episode only for the diagnostic group which covers accidents, injuries, poisoning and violence.

The reasons for this female dominance can be better seen when the rates are broken down in more detail. The illnesses which make the main contribution to the rates under each broad diagnostic heading are shown in Table 6.8. For the moment, we shall leave aside the genito-urinary diseases, pregnancy, and the supplementary classifica-tion. We shall also ignore accidents. General practitioner treatment for accidents and injury in this age group is largely concerned with lacerations, wounds and bruising: men have higher episode rates for each.

Urogenital candidiasis, or thrush, which was not identified at all in earlier GP surveys, is now the most common cause of consultation under *infective and parasitic* diseases for women aged 15–44. How much of the emergence of thrush as a complaint is due to a shift in diagnostic practice, and how much to other factors, such as an

TABLE 6.7   *Rates of episode of GP attention per 1000 at risk, by sex at ages 15–44, for those major diagnostic groups in which the age-specific rate exceeds that of the population: England and Wales 1981–2*

Category	Male		Female	
	15–24	*25–44*	*15–24*	*25–44*
All causes	1270.4	1335.6	2825.3	2728.2
Infectious and parasitic	114.2	88.4	189.9	146.1
Neoplasms	3.7	6.0	7.0	16.7
Endocrine, nutritional and metabolic	7.2	15.4	26.6	42.1
Blood, etc.	1.2	1.3	7.6	13.8
Mental disorders	44.4	80.5	107.3	191.5
Nervous system	90.2	104.6	133.8	147.7
Circulatory	8.9	37.5	16.7	51.3
Respiratory	293.6	263.1	422.2	377.1
Digestive	48.5	71.0	73.2	82.7
Genito-urinary	19.9	22.8	262.1	301.7
Pregnancy, etc.			49.9	40.8
Skin, etc.	150.5	102.9	204.2	147.2
Muscolskeletal	85.9	154.5	103.4	180.5
Signs, symptoms and ill-defined	105.2	116.8	218.3	212.7
Accidents, injury, etc.	194.4	138.4	135.3	115.1
Supplementary classification	100.5	131.5	886.1	660.2

SOURCE: RCGP, 1986

increase in oral contraceptive use, is still not clear. Whatever its source, in our terms candidiasis would qualify as one of those problems associated with the reproductive system, and especially with the female reproductive system. There is only a small difference between the male and female rates for the other major contributor to infective and parasitic problems, which is *intestinal infections*.

Obesity is the main reason for consulting a general practitioner under the heading of *digestive disorders*. Women of all ages are clearly more given to take medical action over obesity then are men, as we saw in an earlier chapter. Men, on the other hand, are more likely to take an active part in sports, and perhaps to make exercise their contribution to weight control. About 35 per cent of men aged 16 and over engage in some outdoor sport or activity, compared with

TABLE 6.8 *Main contributions to a selection of diagnostic groups of GP episodes at ages 15–44: England and Wales 1981–2. Rates per 1000 at risk*

	Male		Female	
Contributory illnesses	15–24	25–44	15–24	25–44
Infectious and parasitic: intestinal; presumed				
infective	30.0	28.2	39.9	30.4
candidiasis	3.2	2.9	49.6	48.3
Digestive:				
obesity	4.3	5.9	20.1	28.4
Mental disorders				
anxiety	11.2	24.3	28.5	59.6
depression	7.1	14.3	31.6	55.3
Nervous system				
conjunctivitis	14.3	14.1	35.3	26.5
earwax	16.3	24.6	14.2	19.4
Respiratory upper respiratory				
tract infection	101.7	165.0	94.0	138.5
tonsillitis	50.7	23.3	85.5	36.3
bronchitis	53.4	35.6	35.8	49.0
catarrh	11.1	12.7	17.1	21.2
hay-fever	33.5	20.1	41.4	26.5
influenza	16.3	24.6	15.2	21.4
asthma	21.9	14.5	18.2	14.6
Skin, etc. other contact				
dermatitis	16.7	15.2	37.7	28.3
acne	37.2	4.8	36.6	11.0
Musculoskeletal				
back-pain	24.6	43.1	28.8	43.1
Signs, symptoms and ill-defined				
headache	11.6	10.2	23.9	22.0
abdominal pains	18.6	19.6	53.5	44.2

SOURCE: RCGP, 1986

21 per cent of women (Birch, 1979). Among the various types of exercise people claim to take, only keep fit/yoga classes and horse-riding are more popular with women, and the numbers involved are very small.

It is, however, difficult to know exactly what the obesity consultations imply. Are women genuinely more likely to be overweight than men? Are women more concerned with their weight than are men? If so, is such a concern based on considerations of female beauty or fashion, or on the pressures of a slimming industry which are primarily directed to women (look at the advertisements in the press); or is it based on a real concern about health?

Alternatively, is it the doctor who is concerned? To put it another way, does the woman herself make the initial approach to a doctor about obesity, or does he raise the topic in the context of a visit for another purpose, such as contraception? Without such information it is impossible to be clear about the underlying causes of women's high rates for this category of consultation.

Almost all of the difference in male and female consultation rates for *blood disorders* results from the diagnosis of iron deficiency anaemia, for which women aged 15–44 have a rate of 10.6 compared to a male rate of 0.5. It is widely believed that anaemia is common among women of childbearing age but there is in fact very little evidence that in Western countries this is true, or that mild anaemia has detrimental effects. After the age of 10, women in general have lower levels of haemoglobin than men, but the levels for both men and women remain stable until extreme old age. 'Anaemia is likely to be used frequently as a "scape-goat" to explain symptoms . . . such as fatigue, breathlessness, dizziness, palpitations and general malaise . . . particularly in women' (Waters and Elwood, 1982). Women using an IUD, or who are pregnant, are also very likely to be tested for, and diagnosed as, anaemic.

It is very difficult to say much about the anxiety and depression which are the main reason for consultations under *mental disorder*. So far as statistics for hospital discharges and deaths from mental disorders go, women aged 15–44 have a slightly lower rate (3.9 per 10 000 population) than men of the same age (4.3 per 10 000). As we saw in Chapter 3, there were tremendous differences between GPs in the classification of mental disorders. As a result, the diagnoses for both sexes are considerably less than satisfactory.

However, in the survey doctors were asked to classify conditions as serious, intermediate or trivial, and we can perhaps assume that the diagnosis of seroius mental disorders is less subject to variation or to whim than the diagnosis of minor conditions (Table 6.9).

Under the classification of *serious mental disorders*, women aged 25–44 have excess rates, although younger women do not. In both age groups the male/female ratios of those diagnosed as having intermediate or trivial mental conditions are similar, but the episode

TABLE 6.9 *GP episode rates per 1000 at risk for categories of mental disorders among those aged 15–44: England and Wales 1981–2*

Category	Male		Female		M/F ratio	
	15–24	*25–44*	*15–24*	*25–44*	*15–24*	*25–44*
Serious	3.3	4.9	3.3	7.5	0.0	0.65
Intermediate	14.1	24.1	41.0	67.9	0.34	0.35
Trivial	27.1	51.5	63.0	116.1	0.43	0.44

SOURCE: RCGP, 1986

rates for women are almost three times higher than for men in the intermediate category, and for trivial disorders more than twice those of men.

Whether there is a genuine difference between the sexes in their reactions to stress, with women becoming anxious or depressed where men resort to drink or aggression is still not clear. It will continue to remain unclear as long as the definitions of stress, and diagnoses of mental conditions, remain confused or even biased by issues of gender discrimination.

From the RCGP report, it appears that there is some overlap in diagnosis between the categories *mental disorder* and *signs, symptoms and ill-defined conditions*. Doctors who describe a large number of patients as mentally ill have few clients about whose signs and symptoms they admit to being baffled. Conversely, doctors who admit to being unable to diagnose quite a large number of conditions describe a much smaller proportion of their patients as suffering from mental illness. To put it another way, some doctors seem prone to consider that any symptom they cannot identify is all in the mind; others simply believe they cannot identify what the complaint implies.

Under the heading of *signs, symptoms and ill-defined* conditions, the quite large contribution of stomach pains should be noted. As we have already seen, women in the reproductive ages with stomach pains are disproportionately likely to be referred to a hospital. However mysterious the cause may be, the pains tend to be a genuine cause of concern to both individual women and to the medical profession.

Women presenting with other ill-diagnosed symptoms, such as headaches, may well be suffering from stress – a condition which, especially in women, requires further exploration. In other instances, the undiagnosed symptoms may represent early signs of disease, particularly of such a disease as multiple sclerosis (more common among women) in which a long latent period may make early diagnosis difficult. The risk of developing multiple sclerosis peaks in the early 30s, although the prevalence in diagnosed cases is higher in later years, and hence it is discussed more fully in the next chapter.

Women aged 15–44 have higher overall rates of GP consultation for *respiratory diseases* then men, but the pattern of different diseases within that group varies quite considerably between the sexes. Men have higher rates of upper respiratory tract infection and influenza, and young men also have more asthma. Women have more tonsillitis, catarrh and hay fever.

Skin problems including dermatitis are more common among women, but young men have marginally higher consultation rates for acne, a reversal of the situation we noted among children.

We can now look at those illnesses and conditions which were earlier put aside: *genito-urinary* diseases, *pregnancy-related conditions*, and those listed under the *supplementary classification* (Table 6.10).

It is immediately evident that these categories of GP episode relate, above all, to reproduction. Vaginal conditions, problems of menstruation, pregnancy and contraception are the reasons for the overwhelming majority of these GP visits.

Many of the visits have nothing to do with illness, as such. Pregnancy diagnosis, prenatal and postpartum care, and a normal delivery; contraceptive advice and supplies; and general health advice are an important part of good preventive medicine, and at least as worthwhile a part of the doctor's functions as treating minor stomach upsets or influenza. If these non-illness consultations are added together, they account for a quarter of all the GP visits by women aged 15–24, and a fifth of those among women aged 25–44.

Statistics on such consultations, while essential for the medical administrator, should *never* be included in any discussion of the morbidity rates of women, or of differential health between men and women.

If we subtract those non-illness consultations from the total rates of GP episodes in Table 6.7 we are left with total rates of 2079 per 1000

TABLE 6.10 *Main contributions to remaining diagnostic groups involving GP episodes in ages 15–44: England and Wales 1981–2. Rates per 1000 at risk*

Contributory condition	Male 15–24	Male 25–44	Female 15–24	Female 25–44
Genito-urinary				
cystitis	5.3	9.9	53.5	55.4
vaginitis			24.6	27.0
premenstrual tension			8.8	30.8
dysmenorrhoea, etc.			30.2	13.3
amenorrhoea, etc.			38.7	22.3
hypermenorrhoea, etc.			24.1	40.9
other genital			19.8	20.4
Pregnancy-related				
abortion, spontaneous			6.8	5.6
abortion, induced			6.4	2.8
haemorrhage in early				
pregnancy			7.1	6.1
delivery			13.2	12.7
Supplementary				
cervical smears			48.8	72.5
general contraceptive				
advice			24.3	16.1
oral contraceptives			369.8	159.6
IUDs			25.1	45.0
letters, certificates,				
etc.	23.6	28.4	31.6	30.9
prenatal care			99.6	78.7
postpartum			52.5	47.1
pregnancy diagnosis			67.3	40.9
advice, health education				
	17.1	17.2	41.1	36.5

SOURCE: RCGP, 1986

women aged 15–24, and 2203 for women aged 25–44. In other words, a woman aged 15–24 may visit a GP with, on average, 2.1 episodes of ill-health, rather than the 2.8 suggested in Table 6.7, and a woman aged 25–44 may have an average of 2.2, rather than 2.7, episodes of ill-health.

A few men also have consultations in the non-illness categories, largely for vasectomy and general health advice, but subtracting these consultations reduces their overall rates of GP episode only marginally, to 1253 per 1000 men aged 15–24, and 1304 for those aged 25–44. Thus, each man's average number of episodes of ill-health would remain virtually unchanged, at about 1.3 for each age-group.

However, even when the non-illness categories are included in the total, it is quite clear that *reproduction is the major factor in the excess GP visits by women* in these age groups. The major contributors alone which are shown in Table 6.10, between them account for 42 per cent of all GP consultations for women aged 15–24, and 37 per cent of those aged 25–44. In other words, if these episodes, which are largely specific to women's reproductive system or related to pregnancy, were excluded, women aged 15–44 would show overall GP episode rates exceeding those of men in the comparable ages by less than 30 per cent, rather than having rates more than double those of men as the crude totals suggest.

Other contributions to the remaining excess come from problems with candidiasis and anaemia, both of which, in this context, could be described as reproductive-related.

The remaining – and comparatively small – causes of illness which produce excess female consultation rates are probably not very important. Some may show up or be raised just because women do visit their doctors for contraception or pregnancy. Others, like ill-defined symptoms and/or mental disorders, may also be linked to physical or emotional problems associated with reproductive issues: until diagnosis is more soundly based, we just will not know.

ILLNESS IN THE COMMUNITY

Sexually transmitted diseases

The statistics from hospital episodes and general practice do not entirely reflect one group of diseases which has its highest incidence among young adults: *sexually transmitted diseases*. This is because a considerable proportion of them are treated in special clinics and so are not included in the figures given above. We have already seen that GPs get a very high incidence of consultation about urogenital candidiasis; the rates for other sexually transmitted diseases are low, but do peak among young adults.

Both men and women aged 15–24 have higher rates of GP visit for genital warts, gonorrhoea, non-specific urethritis (NSU) and tricho-moniasis than do those aged 25–44. Trichomoniasis is largely a problem which women take to a GP; both men and women are almost equally likely to present with genital warts; the rates of GP episode for gonorrhoea and NSU are higher for men.

Sexually transmitted disease clinics in the UK see about 340 000 new cases a year, with about one-third due to NSU (Adler, 1982). Rates for gonorrhoea and syphilis peak in the age-group 20–24 and the same is probably true for other sexually transmitted infections.

Reported ill-health

The Australian Health Survey (ABS, 1986 and ABS, 1986a) gives, as we have seen, further indications of health impairment in the community, by asking about people's illnesses in the fortnight before the survey, and the actions they took for any such illness. Women were more likely to report experience of some illness than men, with 64 per cent of women aged 15–24, and 69 per cent of those aged 25–44, claiming at least one episode of illness compared to 51 and 56 per cent respectively of men in the two age groups.

Among students aged 15–24, a larger proportion of females than males had a day or more away from study (ten per cent of women compared with six per cent of men). Twice as many male students reported one day off as had longer-term illnesses, whereas the girls were evenly divided between those reporting an illness lasting a single day, and longer periods of sickness.

Women aged 15–24 who were working were also more likely to claim to have taken a day off than working men in the same age-group (11 per cent compared with 9 per cent), but about three-fifths of the women only took a single day's leave, while men who took time off for illness were split almost evenly between those who took a single day and those who were off for longer. There was very little difference in the percentages of men and women aged 25–44 who took time off work, or in the amount of time they took: just under half in each sex had a single day's illness.

Consultations with a health professional

Women aged 15–44 were almost twice as likely as men to say that they had consulted a *chemist*. Younger adult men (15–24) were almost twice as likely as women in the same age-group to have seen a *physiotherapist*, presumably because of all those accidents and injuries; the proportions even out in the older age group. Younger adult men were also slightly more likely to have seen a *chiropractor*, but among those aged 25–44 women had the higher number of consultations. There were few consultations with *acupuncturists* by either sex in the 15–24 age group, but women aged 25–44 had consultation levels twice those of men.

Medication

The survey also asked for the types of medication taken in the two weeks prior to interview. Higher percentages of women, in both age groups, had taken painkillers and vitamins or mineral supplements (including, presumably, iron preparations for anaemia); in the other two major categories of medications listed in Table 6.11, men seemed to be more frequent users. Here, as was noted in an earlier chapter, the inclusion of the sex-specific oral contraceptive tends to inflate the total figure for women's use of medicines: two-fifths of the women aged 15–24, and a quarter of those aged 25–44, were using the Pill.

TABLE 6.11 *Percentages of men and women aged 15–44 taking main categories of medication in two weeks prior to survey: Australia 1983*

	Male		Female	
Type(s) of medication	*15–24*	*25–44*	*15–24*	*25–44*
Common pain relievers	47.9	53.4	53.5	86.8
Cough and cold remedies	14.5	10.9	12.1	8.4
Skin ointments/creams	26.5	18.6	18.4	13.2
Vitamin and mineral supplements	36.4	38.6	37.5	45.1
Oral contraceptives			38.5	25.0

SOURCE: ABS, 1986

One reason why women were more likely to report having been ill in the fortnight prior to survey, and why they were more prone to use painkillers, is menstruation. Women aged 15–24 experienced disorders of menstruation at a rate of 23.6 per 1000 and those aged 25–44 had a rate of 29.8. However, because the survey only covered two weeks, the total incidence of menstrual problems over an entire month would be about double those figures.

Menstrual disorders shared seventh place (with influenza) in a list of the most common complaints suffered by *all females of any age* in the sample: had it been possible to analyse the frequency of illnesses only in those age groups affected by menstruation, its ranking would, undoubtedly, have been higher still. Menstrual problems only affect women in their reproductive years, but the Australian Bureau of Statistics did not break down the figures further, simply lumping them in with all complaints at all ages. Here again, one is tempted to conclude that conditions affecting women alone are not given full consideration when the statistics are analysed.

SUMMARY AND CONCLUSIONS

We can sum up the picture of deaths in early adulthood, then, by saying that men have higher death rates at all ages between 15 and 44, and that they also have higher death rates for almost every major cause of death. After age 25, women have significantly higher death rates from only one group of causes – neoplasms. Breast cancer is a major contributor here.

While accidents and suicide do indeed dominate the picture, they cease to be the most important cause of death for men at ages 35–44, and for women at ages 25 and over. It is not merely the difference in the levels of mortality from accident and suicide which account for women's better life expectation in young adulthood. Women's deaths have quite different profile to those of men.

The detailed analysis of illness patterns among young adults shows that the widely held belief that young women have a much higher overall frequency of illness requires considerable modification.

More than 95 per cent of their excess use of hospitals is directly related to their reproductive physiology: their higher hospitalisation rates for neoplasms, because of breast cancer, account for more than the remaining difference. Their apparent very high rate of GP consultation, more than double that of men, is also largely the result of their particular reproductive needs and problems. Subtracting conditions linked to the female reproductive system reduces the excess to 30 per cent; non-illness consultations with a doctor (for pregnancy diagnosis, normal pregnancy, pre- and post-natal care, contraception and general health advice) alone account for a quarter of all consultations by those aged 15–24 and a fifth of all consultations for those aged 25–44.

Self-reporting of illness in the community, which also suggests higher female than male morbidity rates, also turns out, on closer examination, to be biased by definitions of illness and medicines which, in turn, include menstrual problems and the contraceptive Pill.

Nevertheless, when these reproductive factors have been allowed for, it does seem that women aged 15–44 make more use of some health services – especially that of a general practitioner – than do men of the same age. Some of the reasons why they do so are also linked to the reproductive system: consultations for candidiasis, for example. Other conditions may be brought to notice by the doctor himself, when the woman visits for another purpose such as contraception: some of the episodes of varicose veins, anaemia and obesity, for example, may fall into such a category. A third group, covering many of the conditions which some GPs diagnose as mental problems and others as signs, symptoms and ill-defined conditions, is, by its very nature, vague and requires more thorough study that it has yet been given.

Are women presenting with vague symptoms because of a greater health awareness? Do the symptoms result from stress, and if so do women face greater, or different, stresses than men – or do they simply react to stress in a different way? Too much should not be made of this residual problem, which is quite small in this age group. (The situation is different in those aged over 45, and will be considered more extensively in the next chapter.) The combined rates of general practitioner consultations for mental problems plus 'signs, symptoms and ill-defined conditions' account for 11 per cent of both male and female diagnoses at ages 15–24, and 15 per cent of male and female diagnoses at ages 25–44. Perhaps a part of the answer is that modern medicine cannot offer a good diagnosis for a small percentage of patients, whatever their sex!

7 Health in the Middle and Later Years

'Middle age' is one of those flexible phrases which we all use as we prefer. To an adolescent, parents – even parents below the age of forty – are already middle aged; to an 85-year-old mother, a son in his sixties is probably just approaching middle age.

To some extent, definitions of middle and old age depend on total life expectation. In a country where the average expectation of life is only around sixty years, somebody in his or her fifties is quite elderly. China's life expectation is now ten years above that, but the change has been so recent that the Chinese still describe middle age as beginning at 35, while old age is synonymous with retirement, at 55 for women and 60 for men. In the industrialised world, by contrast, most of us can expect to live at least into our seventies. We have pushed back the frontiers of middle and old age.

Most of the statistics we shall be dealing with in this chapter divide people into the age-groups 45–64; 65–74; and 75 and above. So it seems reasonable to describe those *aged 45–64 as middle aged*, and those *over 75 as the very old*.

Those *aged 65–74* are the difficulty. Many are as fit and active as the middle-aged. Some, retired from work but busy in the garden and with a host of other activities, may be fitter than their younger friends, in the sense that they take more exercise and eat more sensibly than is often possible for somebody in a job. Others have already developed the kind of health profile seen more commonly in the very old: they may suffer from a range of chronic diseases and disabilities and be able only to enjoy a very restricted life. Although the 65–74 group will be described, simply for convenience, as *the old*, the fact that they are a very disparate group should never be forgotten.

DEATH RATES IN MIDDLE AGE

Death rates for both men and women begin to increase quite sharply once they reach their mid forties. By around age fifty, however, there is an increasingly obvious divergence between male and female survival chances. Male death rates in England and Wales, for example, rise so much more swiftly than those of women that women aged 60–64 have lower death rates than men five years younger (Table 7.1). In Australia the level of mortality of women aged 45–49 is about the same of males aged 40–44. The gap widens with increasing age, so that at 60–65 women have levels of mortality similar to those of men seven years younger.

TABLE 7.1 *Death rates per 1000, by sex, for those aged 45–64:*
England and Wales 1984

Age	Male	Female
45–49	3.99	2.52
50–54	7.05	4.31
55–59	12.66	7.29
60–64	21.57	11.49

SOURCE: OPCS, 1986d

CAUSES OF DEATH IN MIDDLE AGE

The most common causes of death in the middle years are, for both sexes, *cancers* and *heart diseases*. Between them, they account for approximately two-thirds of all deaths at ages 45–64. However, the importance of each of these two major causes of death is rather different for men and women, and at different ages (Table 7.2).

In the age group 45–54, deaths from diseases of the *circulatory system* predominate among men, while for women *cancers* are the major cause of death. Among those aged 55–64, while that overall difference remains, it is less marked. *Cancers* become increasingly significant as a cause of male, and *circulatory system* diseases a cause of female, deaths.

Cancers

There are, of course, a variety of cancers, and by the time men and women reach the middle years they are becoming susceptible to most

TABLE 7.2   *Major causes of death at ages 45–64, by sex: England, Rates per 100 000 population*

| Cause | Male | | | Female | |
	45–54	55–64		45–54	55–64
All causes	542.5	1700.7		335.3	941.9
Neoplasms	162.2	568.6		183.5	434.4
Circulatory system	266.8	862.6		77.5	328.5
Respiratory	20.6	105.9		14.5	58.3
Digestive	17.2	42.4		12.6	28.7
Injury and poisoning	45.8	47.5		22.2	27.6

SOURCE: OPCS, 1968d

of them. However, lung cancer and cancer of the breast, for men and women respectively, are overwhelmingly the most significant as causes of death in these age-groups.

Lung cancer and cancer of the trachea and bronchus account for 31 per cent of male cancer deaths at ages 45–54, and for 40 per cent of male cancer deaths at ages 55–64. By contrast, they account for only 12 and 19 per cent of female deaths in the two age groups respectively.

Women are more likely to die from breast cancer, which is the cause of 35 per cent of all cancer deaths to women aged 45–54, and a quarter of all cancer deaths in the ages 55–64.

Other frequent types of cancer include the sex-specific cancers of the cervix and uterus, and of the prostate. Cervical and uterine cancer combined produce death rates of 116 per million in the women aged 45–54 and 270 among those aged 55–64. Cancer of the prostate lead to a death rate of 22 for each million men aged 45–54, and 197 for those aged 55–64. In other words, women aged 45–54 are almost six times more likely to die from genital cancers than are men, while at ages 55–64 the male rates have increased to a level around two-thirds that of women.

Women in both age groups show substantially lower death rates from each of the remaining types of cancer than do men. In most instances, their death rates were only around half those of men.

Thus the vulnerability of women aged 45–64 to death from cancer is largely a vulnerability to cancers of the breast, cervix and uterus. Men have higher death rates not merely from lung cancer, but from all other malignancies. Cancers may have the greatest prominence as the cause of death for women 45–64, but in fact women in those age groups are less likely overall to die from cancer than men, and their deaths are concentrated in a small group of types of cancer.

Circulatory system

The female health advantage is even more apparent when deaths from diseases of the *circulatory system* are considered. Women aged 45–54 have death rates from these diseases which are less than a third those of men; even in the age group 55–64, female death rates are well below half those of men.

The specific causes of death under this diagnostic heading are also rather different for the two sexes. The vast majority – eighty per cent – of the male deaths at ages 45–54 are due to ischaemic heart disease while only half of the female deaths are from this cause. The much greater mortality rate for men means that their actual *risk* of death from ischaemic heart disease is about five times that of women. At ages 55–64 the gap narrows slightly, with 78 per cent of male, and 59 per cent of female, deaths from diseases of the circulatory system being due to ischaemic heart disease: this still produces a male risk of death which is three times greater than that of women.

For both sexes, most of the remaining deaths from diseases of the circulatory system are from cerebrovascular disease. That implies, of course, that although women's death rates from cerebrovascular disease are below those of men, a larger *proportion* of all female deaths are due to this cause.

To put it another way, the very much larger risk which men aged 45–64 have of dying of some disease of the circulatory system is almost entirely due to their being more prone to ischaemic heart disease. The risks of men and women dying from other circulatory diseases, expressed as a rate per million, are much more equal.

Respiratory diseases

Women have death rates from *respiratory diseases* which are about half those of men. Almost two-thirds of the female deaths are from bronchitis, emphysema and asthma, while only two-fifths of male deaths are from those causes.

Digestive diseases

The differences between male and female death rates from diseases of the *digestive system* are smaller, although here too women do better. The specific causes of death are quite similar for each sex; the overall female advantage does not seem to result from any difference in the types of digestive disease they get, but simply from a lower overall incidence. Chronic liver disease and cirrhosis of the liver account for about half of the risk of death, for each sex, from digestive diseases. Another important contribution – again for both sexes – comes from duodenal and stomach ulcers.

Injury and poisoning

Men in the age groups 45–64 continue to have more *accidents and injuries* than women, but the gap between death rates for each sex is smaller than in the earlier years, and declines with increasing age. While men aged 45–54 have accident rates around double those of women, among those aged 55–64 the excess is somewhat less. Accidents involving a motor vehicle are far less common among women than men, especially in the age group 45–54. Male car-accident rates at this age are almost twice those fo women.

To some extent these differences may result from differential car use between the sexes, although they may also reflect different driving behaviour. Australia, despite having far more widespread car ownership than is the case in England and Wales, and a much greater use by women of cars, also produces male car-accident rates which are double those of women in the age groups 45–54.

DEATH IN THE LATER YEARS

The difference between male and female death rates continues to be very large at ages 65–69; women's death rates are still only just over half those of men. With increasing age thereafter, the difference gradually declines, although it remains quite substantial until ages above ninety (Table 7.3).

TABLE 7.3   *Death rates per 1000, by sex for those aged 65–99: England and Wales 1984*

Age	Male	Female	M/F ratio
65–69	35.00	18.44	1.90
70–74	54.46	29.15	1.87
75–79	84.64	48.31	1.76
80–84	129.89	82.14	1.58
85–89	191.55	139.37	1.37
90–94	272.01	226.99	1.20
95–99	298.49	285.75	1.04

SOURCE: OPCS, 1986d

CAUSES OF DEATH IN THE LATER YEARS

The major causes of death for those aged 65 and above are broadly similar to those for people aged 45–64. Deaths from diseases of the *circulatory system* and from *cancer* predominate, followed by those

TABLE 7.4   *Major causes of death at ages 65–85+, by sex: England and Wales 1984 Rates per 100 000 population.*

Cause	Male			Female		
	65–74	75–84	85+	65–74	75–84	85+
All causes	4400.2	9928.4	21159.4	2378.1	6163.8	16883.9
Neoplasms	1343.7	2353.6	3171.8	757.0	1163.8	1745.3
Endocrine, nutritional, etc.	46.5	134.6	263.9	45.5	121.8	257.3
Mental disorders	34.7	188.1	618.4	27.9	172.3	741.3
Nervous system	64.8	198.8	419.5	41.4	117.0	261.5
Circulatory system	2240.0	4987.3	10352.2	1150.7	3472.8	9523.2
Respiratory	418.5	1370.7	4243.0	160.8	520.5	2442.1
Digestive	99.8	252.4	608.6	77.6	225.7	630.6
Genito-urinary	39.1	169.8	650.2	25.1	104.4	311.8
Injury and poisoning	67.2	131.6	313.5	45.5	108.7	309.7

SOURCE OPCS, 1986d

from diseases of the *respiratory* and *digestive* systems and from *accidents*. However, in these older age groups cancer ceases to be the most important cause of female deaths. Instead, women join men in diseases of the circulatory system as the principle underlying cause of death (Table 7.4).

Circulatory system

The male risk of death from diseases of the *circulatory system* at ages 65–74 continues to be almost twice that of women. At older ages, however, the difference narrows quite rapidly.

The most important cause of death under this heading is ischaemic heart disease. It accounts for almost half the female deaths from diseases of the circulatory system at ages 65–85, and for more than half the male deaths. Thus the advantage in lower mortality from ischaemic heart disease which was shown by women in the younger age groups is reduced quite rapidly in old age.

Most of the remaining deaths from diseases of the circulatory system, for both sexes, are from cerebro-vascular disease. The rates for men are a little higher than those for women at each age until age 85. Hypertension is the third most common cause of death in this group, and here too male rates are somewhat higher until ages 85 and over.

By contrast, women have substantially higher death rates than men from chronic rheumatic heart disease at all ages, and their rates are three times as high at ages 85 and above.

Cancers

Cancers of the lung, trachea and bronchus continue to account for about 40 per cent of all male deaths from cancer in the ages 65–74. After that their importance begins to decrease, with about one-third of cancer deaths at ages 75–84, and a quarter of those at ages 85 and over, being due to these causes. Among women aged 65–74, cancers of the lung, trachea and bronchus begin to become important as a cause of death; they account for a fifth of the female deaths from cancer in that age group. Among women of older ages, however, these types of cancer are less significant. The women aged 65–74 were born in 1910–20, and presumably started smoking around the time of the Second World War.

Breast cancer among women aged 65 and over declines in its proportional importance: it accounts for rather less than a fifth of the female deaths from cancer.

Deaths from cancer of the prostate contribute about eight per cent to male cancer deaths at ages 65–74, and this proportion rises to one-fifth at ages 85 and above. About seven per cent of deaths of women aged 65–74 are from cervical and uterine cancer; in the older age groups the percentage falls still further.

For most of the remaining common cancers, men at all ages above 65 show considerably higher death rates than women. The difference is greatest for cancer of the bladder, where the death rate for women is only a third of the male rate, and smallest for colonic cancer, where women have rates 80 per cent those of men.

Respiratory

Males have considerably higher rates of death than females from diseases of the *respiratory system*. At ages 65–75, about a third of female, and more than a third of male, deaths are due to bronchitis, emphysema and asthma. With increasing age, pneumonia becomes more important as a cause until, at ages 85 and over, it accounts for over half of the male, and four-fifths of the female, deaths.

The high incidence of deaths from pneumonia at very old ages may not truly reflect the actual risk of the disease as an underlying cause of death. In most cases, pneumonia in the elderly follows upon some other cause – an episode of influenza, for example, or a bad fall. Under the International Classification of Diseases principles, such deaths should be attributed to the underlying cause. In other words, the disease or injury which starts the biological process leading, ultimately, to death is the one which should appear in the statistics. It is probable that, where such a large proportion of deaths among the very old is described as due to pneumonia, many should really have been classified elsewhere. However, it should be pointed out that, among very old people with several health impairments it is often difficult to identify which one *was* the underlying cause.

Digestive diseases

Among those aged 65 and over, stomach and duodenal ulcers are responsible for a high proportion of the deaths from diseases of the digestive system. The death rates are higher among men than women until age 85, when they become more or less equal. Chronic liver disease and cirrhosis decrease in importance as a cause of death in each age group, but the male rates always remain considerably above those of women.

Injuries and poisoning

The male dominance in death rates from *injuries and poisoning* decreases with age until, at 85 years and over, the rates are almost identical for men and women. Men continue to have twice the rate of death from motor accidents at all ages, but these become increasingly less important as a cause of death. They give way to accidental falls, which become the major cause of death under this heading. At ages 75–84 and, more particularly, after age 85, women have a higher death rate from falls than do men.

Suicide is another factor in the levels of mortality from injuries and poisoning. As was discussed in the previous chapter, suicide rates increase with age so that, although the absence of many other causes of death among young people makes the contribution of suicide to their death rates very noticeable, it is the elderly who are more likely to kill themselves. This is particularly the case for males, as Figure 7.1 shows.

Males over the age of 70 have the highest suicide rates of all ages, both for men and women. By contrast, suicide rates for women peak at about 70 and decline thereafter (Bulusu and Alderton, 1984).

Other causes of death

The great majority of deaths under the classification endocrine, nutritional, etc. are due to diabetes mellitus. For both sexes this becomes a quite significant cause of death after age 75. Rates are slightly lower for women at all ages.

The statistics used here contain no further breakdown of the causes of death under *mental disorders*; we shall simply note, at this point in the chapter, that men have higher rates at all ages to 85 years.

Neither is there a more detailed breakdown for the causes of death from diseases of the nervous system; here too we shall simply note, for the present, that the death rates at each age are quite substantially higher for males.

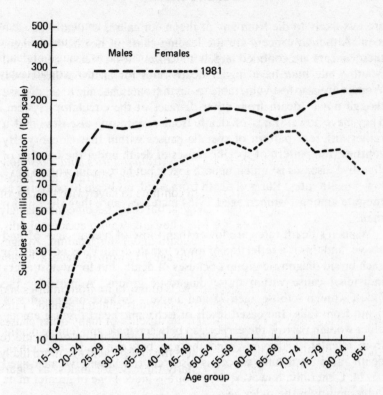

Figure 7.1   Age-specific suicide rates, by sex: England and Wales, 1981.
SOURCE: Bulusu and Alderton, 1984.

Genito-urinary diseases do not figure largely among the causes of death at ages 65–74, but they become important amongst the older population. About two-thirds of the deaths in this broad category at ages 65–74, and around half of those at 85 and above, are due to kidney inflammations. Among males, most of the remaining deaths result from enlargement of the prostate.

TRENDS AND PATTERNS OF DEATHS IN MIDDLE AND OLD AGE

We can sum up these figures by concluding that women's death rates at ages 45–64 rise much less sharply than do those of men. Women are less likely to die from any of the major causes of death than are men. Although cancers are the leading cause of death for women, their cancers are confined largely to cancer of the breast, cervix and womb while men have higher death rates for all the other types. Women are also less vulnerable to death from ischaemic heart disease though not to death from other diseases of the circulatory system. They have lower rates of death from respiratory diseases, and a rather different pattern of specific causes within that category. By contrast, the pattern of specific causes of death under the heading of digestive diseases is similar in both sexes, but here again women have lower death rates. Rates of death from accidents begin to converge as the rate amongst women aged 55–64 increases more than the rate for men.

Women's death rates are lower than those of men at ages 65 and above, and this is a reflection of lower female death rates not only for each broad diagnostic group of causes of death, but for almost every individual cause within those diagnostic groups. Admittedly, the oldest women – those aged 75 and above – do have higher rates of death from falls. Increased levels of ischaemic heart disease among older women narrow the earlier gap between male and female deaths from circulatory diseases, and the gap between male and female death rates from lung cancer is also reduced among women aged 65–74. Generally, however, the picture is indeed one of greater male vulnerability in the older ages.

Male high death rates from lung cancer at comparatively early ages form a major contribution to the overall large excess in male death rates in middle life. Were it not for the rather high female death rates during the same ages from breast cancer, the gap between male and female longevity would be still greater. However, in recent years women have shown increasing death rates from lung cancer, while the rates for men have actually declined.

Cigarette smoking, atmospheric pollution and occupational exposure are all thought to be factors in the development of lung cancer. The increase in female death rates is associated with increased smoking among women – especially during and since the Second World War – while declines in male death rates, especially at the younger ages, are thought to result from declines in cigarette smoking and an increased preference for mild and filter-tipped cigarettes. It is possible that this explains the comparatively high death rates from cancer for women aged 65–74, which are not matched in older women. Women aged 65–74 in 1984 were probably the first generation of women for whom cigarette smoking was acceptable, and this could be a factor in the increase in female deaths. If subsequent generations of women have indeed become more vulnerable to smoking-related deaths, we could see increased female mortality rates reducing the gap between female and male life expectation in future.

However, there are differences in levels of mortality from lung cancer between countries, and differences in the sex ratio of deaths, which are still unexplained (Kazantzis, 1982). Nevertheless, it is clear that many deaths from lung cancer, especially at comparatively young ages, could be prevented and that the effect on life expectation would be considerable.

The incidence of breast cancer, which results in a high proportion of women's deaths in the age groups 45–64, seems to have been increasing in recent decades, not only in England and Wales but elsewhere in the Western world. Unfortunately, the origins of breast cancer are less understood than those of cancer of the lung and thus prevention is more difficult. Widespread screening of women at five-yearly intervals, and early treatment, might reduce the death rate, at least among younger women (Chamberlain, 1982a; 1984). However, as childless women appear to have a greater risk of breast cancer, trends towards an increasing proportion of women who choose to remain childless could increase the incidence.

Elderly women appear to be particularly vulnerable to deaths resulting from accidental falls. One reason is that they live often alone. They are more likely to be widowed than a man of comparable age, and are less likely to be living with other family members. A survey in 1976 of the elderly in England (Hunt, 1978) found that nearly 40 per cent of women aged 75–84 lived alone, and more than half of those aged 85 and over. Comparable percentages for men were 15, and less than 30.

Old people may also lack satisfactory housing and other amenities which might help them to avoid an accident, or get assistance if one occurs. The same survey reported that 'possession of many things which younger people would consider essential for satisfactory living shows a marked decline with increasing age' so that those aged 85 and above were the least likely to have a bathroom, inside lavatory, hot water supply, or telephone, for example.

In one sense, the mortality statistics which we have been looking at come as no surprise. Given that men die, on the whole, earlier than women, it is inevitable that, at most ages, their death rates for a variety of diseases are higher. Given that the earlier deaths of men are widely suspected to be connected with a male lifestyle, it is not surprising to find that many of those deaths are from diseases which are linked to personal behaviour. Higher levels of smoking, consumption of alcohol, (mis)use of cars, and so on obviously play a part in these excess deaths.

In another sense, however, the figures do come as a surprise. The higher male death rates at most ages, not merely in almost every broad category of diseases but from almost every major cause of death within each category, suggest that there is a widespread male vulnerability which leads men either to more illness, or to succumb to illnesses at an earlier stage of life. Whether middle-aged and elderly men have more illness, or whether they simply have more fatal illness, an examination of other health statistics may help to determine.

HOSPITAL EPISODES

The figures for hospital discharges (including deaths) in England in 1984 reveal rather more complex patterns of hospital use by sex among the middle-aged and elderly population than was the case in the younger age groups. One thing which is immediately noticeable is that the durations of stay in hospital increase quite rapidly for both women and men after they reach their mid forties. Up to that age, most hospital episodes involve stays of less than a week but from 45 years onwards, and particularly after age 65, a stay in hospital tends to be a comparatively long occurrence (Table 7.5).

During the reproductive years, as the previous chapter indicated, women had higher hospital discharge rates and higher average daily use of beds. Women aged 45–49 continue to outnumber men in those statistics, but their proportionate use of hospitals declines during the next five-year period. At ages above 55, men have higher discharge rates and use more hospital beds.

After age 50, however, women who are in hospital tend to be there for a longer stay than men of the same age. The difference is most marked at ages 60–64. This longer duration of stay in hospital by older women may reflect the higher proportion of male hospital episodes which end in death. However, it may also reflect the need to provide convalescent care for those women who live alone or with an elderly husband.

TABLE 7.5   *Hospital discharges (including deaths) at ages 45–64: England 1984*

Category	45–49	50–54	50–59	60–64
Discharge rates per 10000 population				
male	747.4	932.3	1186.2	1464.0
female	980.6	968.2	958.8	1059.9
ratio m/	0.76	0.96	1.24	1.38
Average number of beds used daily per million population				
male	1959	2700	3847	5082
female	2553	3103	3263	4781
ratio m/f	0.77	0.87	1.18	1.06
Mean duration of stay (days)				
male	7.3	8.3	9.4	9.8
female	7.3	9.2	9.5	11.5

SOURCE: DHSS, 1986

The Report of the Hospital In-Patient Enquiry does not provide a detailed age breakdown of the causes of hospital episodes. Instead, it groups together all those aged 45–64. Table 7.6 shows diseases of the female genital organs as the second most common cause of a hospital episode for women in these age groups. Gynaecological conditions, and problems associated with the menopause, probably account for much of the female excess hospital use at ages 45–49. In later years, these reproductive-related conditions give way to an increasing incidence of malignant or benign neoplasms.

Women aged 45–64 also have marginally higher rates of hospital episode for *endocrine and nutritional* conditions, diseases of the *nervous system*, and *musculoskeletal* conditions.

Despite women's higher hospitalisation rates under those five headings, the table shows that for most major diseases the male rate of hospital episodes is higher than that of women. In other words, women aged 45–64 are less likely than men to be hospitalised for most other conditions.

The suggestion already made that diseases of the *genital organs* are probably most frequently found among the women aged 45–49 is

TABLE 7.6 *Discharges and deaths in hospital at ages 45–64, by sex and major diagnostic group, per 10 000 population: England 1984*

Diagnosis	Male	Female
All causes	1801.3	993.6
Neoplasms	140.1	173.9
Endocrine, nutritional, etc.	18.8	21.8
Nervous system	21.9	22.6
Ischaemic heart disease	119.4	34.4
Acute myocardial infarction	60.4	17.5
Pulmonary and other heart	36.2	20.5
Cerebrovascular	26.2	16.6
Other circulatory	53.8	44.5
Respiratory	67.9	44.5
Other digestive	133.6	84.6
Urinary	31.2	19.0
Male genital organs	32.8	
Female genital organs		145.9
Musculoskeletal	66.8	81.9
Injury and poisoning	74.3	59.0
Signs, symptoms and ill-defined	162.1	131.2

SOURCE DHSS, 1986

confirmed, to some extent, by a closer look at the figures. Under this heading, the female complaints include pelvic inflammatory disease, inflammatory diseases of the womb, and menstrual disorders.

The neoplasms which lead to women's higher rates of hospitalisation under this heading are divided into malignant and benign or unspecified. They involve predominantly neoplasms of the breast and uterus. The hospital discharge rate for malignant neoplasms, or cancers, of the breast and uterus are 35.0 and 15.1 per 10 000, respectively. Benign and unspecified neoplasms of the uterus produce a hospital discharge rate of 18.2 per 10 000.

So far as other common neoplasms are concerned, men in these age groups have almost twice the female rate for lung cancer, and almost four times the rate for cancer of the bladder.

It is difficult to identify why women have slightly higher overall rates of hospitalisation under the heading *endocrine, nutritional, etc.*, as the figures are not broken down in sufficient detail. Diabetes mellitus is the major condition shown; it accounts for two-thirds of the male hospitalisation rate under this heading but only half of the female rate.

One contribution to the higher female rate of hospital discharge for diseases of the central *nervous system* is multiple sclerosis. Although the disease most commonly develops in the thirties, prevalence rates are highest between ages 40 and 65 and women are affected more frequently than men, with a ratio of 3:2 (Shelley and Dean, 1982). There is a genetic predisposition to this disease.

Among the *musculoskeletal* problems, arthropathies – diseases of the joints – are the most likely to result in hospital treatment. Of these, rheumatoid arthritis, at least, does appear to have a sex ratio which is higher for women (Wood and Badley, 1982).

When we turn to the older population aged 65 and over, the male domination of discharge rates which started at ages 55–59 can be seen to continue in each age group. In other words, men use hospitals more frequently than women at all ages above 54 (Table 7.7).

However, we noted that women aged 50 and over who were hospitalised tended to occupy those beds for a longer period. This trend intensifies among older women, whose duration of stay is

TABLE 7.7 *Hospital discharges (including deaths) at ages 65 and above: England 1984*

Catagory	65–69	70–74	75–79	80–84	85–89	90+
Discharge rates per 1000 population						
male	1841.3	2391.6	2997.7	3651.7	4594.4	
female	1324.8	1631.6	2091.9	2681.2	3660.5	
ratio m/f	1.39	1.47	1.43	1.36	1.26	
Average number of beds used daily per million pop,						
male	5748	7851	7503	5807	2845	1441
female	5884	10119	12958	14926	11291	6534
ratio m/f	0.98	0.78	0.58	0.39	0.25	0.22
Mean duration of stay						
male	12.4	14.1	19.0	20.2	24.5	31.3
female	14.5	19.6	24.0	32.7	39.8	45.0

SOURCE: DHSS, 1986

increasingly longer than that of men in every five-year age group. Here again, one reason for women's longer stay in hospital is that a man's stay is more likely to end in his death. But the fact that the divergence in length of stay increases so sharply after the age of 70 also suggests that women may be kept in hospital longer because of a lack of convalescent support at home.

A man in his 70s, or even older, is much more likely than a woman of the same age to have a spouse. If he does, it is also likely that his wife will be reasonably active, because men generally marry women a few years younger than themselves. Conversely, a woman in her early 70s is more likely to be a widow, and, even where she has a living husband, he is likely to be very elderly and perhaps not capable of providing much nursing care. Elderly single, widowed or divorced women are also more likely than men in the same situation to be living alone; a point which is discussed in more detail later on.

A different profile of disease between the two sexes may also help to explain the different length of stay in hospital, and this can be examined in Table 7.8

The figures for most of the causes of an episode in hospital follow the pattern that one would expect: that is, they rise steadily in each of the three age groups, so that those aged 85+ have the highest rates of hospital use for almost all causes. There are, however, a few exceptions to the pattern of increases in all conditions over time.

Men and women are most likely to be hospitalised for *cancers* between ages 75 and 84. With increasing age, both men and women fall victim to an increasingly wide range of cancers so that, while neoplasms of the lung, bladder and (in women) breast and womb continue to be major causes of illness and death, they no longer dominate the statistics so forcefully. Men aged 75–84 also have peak rates for acute myocardial infarction – coronary thrombosis – and diseases of the male genital organs, mostly enlarged prostate. By contrast, diseases of the female genital organs, which were so important a cause of hospitalisation for women aged 45–64, decrease steadily with age.

The other immediately obvious pattern in Table 7.8 is one of higher male hospital discharge rates at every age from almost every cause. There are only three causes of a hospital stay for which women have higher rates, but those rates are higher at all ages from 65: they are *mental disorders*, *musculoskeletal* diseases, and *injury* and *poisoning*.

TABLE 7.8 *Discharge and deaths in hospital at ages 65–85+, by sex and major diagnostic group, per 10 000 population: England 1984*

Diagnosis	Male 65–74	75–84	85+	Female 65–74	75–84	85+
All causes	2016.4	3216.1	4594.4	1481.4	2326.1	3660.5
Neoplasms	395.3	542.4	524.0	249.1	260.0	230.5
Mental disorders	12.4	41.6	106.0	13.0	48.7	119.8
Nervous system	49.1	84.0	111.5	36.4	62.2	72.5
Ischaemic heart	159.1	179.3	180.3	79.1	120.7	141.0
Acute myocardial infarction	104.5	121.5	109.1	48.3	80.9	84.8
Pulmonary and other heart	101.0	205.9	336.7	67.7	141.3	265.7
Cerebrovascular	92.3	180.3	289.5	62.4	150.9	255.7
Respiratory	177.0	348.5	646.3	87.8	150.8	322.1
Pneumonia	31.2	102.3	281.0	17.8	54.7	164.8
Other digestive	210.6	299.3	382.4	140.3	215.6	293.9
Urinary	68.9	93.1	158.7	30.6	41.4	57.3
Male genital organs	105.8	139.5	132.4			
Female genital organs				62.4	44.2	27.7
Musculoskeletal	86.6	94.7	136.2	118.7	144.1	195.1
Injury and poisoning	79.8	139.4	343.7	107.2	252.9	549.8
Signs, symptoms and ill-defined	275.2	414.7	593.7	175.0	280.1	460.0

SOURCE: DHSS, 1986

Without a more detailed breakdown of the *mental disorders*, it is difficult to find reasons for the female excess, which is very small at ages 65–74, but increases in the oldest age groups. It may be that elderly women are genuinely more likely to suffer severe mental illness. Alternatively, the difference in hospital use could result from, or be augmented by, a lack of family support for elderly women at home.

About half of the hospital episodes for both men and women in each age group which are caused by *musculoskeletal* problems, are for arthropathies – diseases of the joints. Probably the main reason why women have higher rates of musculoskeletal illness is that in old age they are more likely to suffer from osteoporosis, or an increasing porousness of bone. As Table 7.6 showed, women in the middle years already begin to have higher rates of hospital episode for musculoskeletal conditions, although the difference in rates between men and women increases noticeably in old age. Changes in the female hormone balance after the menopause are thought to be responsible for women's particular vulnerability to this aspect of ageing.

Osteoporosis may also help to explain the higher female injury rates among the hospital discharges. Fractures account for 54 per cent of hospital episodes under this heading among women aged 65–74, and among women aged 85 and over the percentage with a fracture rises to 70. Fractures are a less important contributor to the male injury rates, at 35 per cent for men aged 65–74, and 56 per cent for those aged 85 and above. Among the fractures which bring both men and women to hospital, a break of the neck of the femur (a fractured hip) is the most common.

These three causes of a hospital episode do, perhaps, go some way towards explaining the longer stays in hospital by women. While they may be less dramatic than a coronary episode, for example, they tend to be comparatively long-term to treat.

With these exceptions, it is apparent that both sexes are hospitalised for much the same reasons, but that men of each age group have much higher rates. In other words, men in the older age groups seem to have a greater vulnerability to almost the whole range of illnesses and causes of death, and their greater vulnerability is apparent at earlier ages.

The picture of overall illness and death for those aged 45 and over, as measured by hospital use, suggests that women from the age of 55 have lower discharge rates and lower bed use than men. The fact that women who do spend time in hospital remain there longer than men is partly a reflection of the higher rates of male death. It is also partly the result of a different pattern of illness between the sexes, and different prospects of home care for elderly men and women.

Until the end of their reproductive period women continue to be hospitalised rather frequently for gynaecological conditions. In their 50s and 60s, high rates of breast and uterine cancer are a major cause of illness and death, but otherwise the reasons for a hospital stay are not very different between the sexes. In old age, women have higher rates of hospitalisation for mental disorders, musculoskeletal problems, and injuries – especially fractures. Men have higher rates of hospital discharge for the majority of complaints at all ages from 45 onwards; they appear to be more prone to almost all serious illnesses, as well as to death.

ILLNESS AS SEEN BY THE GENERAL PRACTITIONER

The survey of general practitioner practices in England and Wales (RCGP, 1986) divides the age groups of patients in a similar way to the Hospital In-patient Enquiry (Table 7.9). However, it does not separate the old from the very old, but simply combines all those above age 75. Nevertheless, so long as it is kept in mind that much of the reported illness is probably concentrated in the later years, this grouping should not affect our examination of the sex patterns of illness at different stages of life.

TABLE 7.9   *Rates of episode of GP attention, per 1000 at risk by sex, at ages 45 and above, for most important diagnostic groups; England and Wales 1981–2*

Category	Male			Female		
	45–64	65–74	75+	45–64	65–74	75+
All causes	1648.7	2143.3	2612.1	2291.6	2440.4	2738.5
Mental disorders	97.8	86.6	110.0	202.2	187.5	190.2
Nervous system	136.8	189.2	218.6	166.5	184.1	211.7
Circulatory	181.0	364.2	450.3	180.6	347.7	428.9
Respiratory	249.2	356.1	397.6	319.2	305.8	272.6
Digestive	97.1	131.0	163.4	103.4	131.7	142.1
Genito-urinary	33.4	62.6	92.6	175.5	81.4	81.9
Skin, etc.	100.2	116.7	121.5	121.3	130.0	132.2
Musculoskeletal	226.6	237.8	236.3	295.4	330.0	347.2
Signs, symptoms and ill-defined	145.2	204.5	313.7	208.7	260.5	365.4
Accidents, injury, etc	112.6	89.7	107.9	126.1	136.9	179.8

SOURCE: RCGP, 1986

The division between the sexes in illness as seen by a general practitioner is very different to that seen in hospitals. Women appear to dominate the statistics, although there are some shifts in the pattern at different ages.

The rates of GP consultation tend to rise in every age group, as one would expect. For men, the exceptions are treatments for *musculoskeletal* conditions, which stabilise in the older ages, and for *accidents and injuries* which are highest in the 45–64 age group. Women, on the other hand, have steadily declining rates of GP episode at each age group for *respiratory* diseases and *genito-urinary* diseases, and a drop in *mental disorders* after age 65.

At ages 45–64, women have higher rates of GP consultation for all major causes. Their excess is particularly marked for *mental disorders* and *genito-urinary diseases*, and – to a somewhat lesser extent – for *respiratory* and *musculoskeletal* conditions, and diseases of the *nervous system*. They also dominate the residual category of *signs, symptoms and ill-defined conditions*.

Cystitis is the major contributor to the excesss female rate of genito-urinary complaint at ages 45–64. With increasing age, male rates of cystitis rise markedly while those of women do not; older men also develop prostate problems.

Respiratory conditions, to which women seem so much more prone in the ages 45–64, are, when looked at in more detail, made up largely of higher rates for respiratory tract infections, sinusitis, tonsillitis, laryngitis, bronchitis, catarrh, asthma and hay-fever. Men have higher rates for influenza, chronic bronchitis and emphysema: the latter two being possibly associated with environmental conditions or life-style behaviour such as smoking.

Diseases of the central *nervous system* include multiple sclerosis and migraine, where the rates of GP consultation are three times as high for women aged 45–64 as men.

As was briefly mentioned earlier, multiple sclerosis occurs more frequently in females, with a ratio of 3:2. Women also tend to develop it earlier, and, while the risk is highest in the thirties, the difficulty of establishing a diagnosis means that the reported prevalence is greatest at around age 50. There is a genetic component to multiple sclerosis, with immediate relatives having a risk of acquiring it which is considerably above the risk in the population as a whole (Shelley and Dean, 1982).

Migraine is also known to be much more common in women than men. It may be the result of a specific biochemical deficiency, and may involve a genetic predisposition. It often begins at puberty, and may disappear during pregnancy or with the menopause.,

After age 65, women have higher rates of GP episode for only half of the major causes of consultation listed in Table 7.9. These are *mental disorders*, *skin* problems, *musculoskeletal* conditions, *accidents and injuries* and *signs, symptoms and ill-defined* conditions.

The major complaint under *skin problems* is contact dermatitis, where the rates for both sexes are very similar.

Just about every condition listed under *musculoskeletal* diseases shows higher female than male rates. Particularly noticeable are the differences in rheumatoid arthritis and arthritis, where women's rates are almost double those of men. As was noted earlier in the chapter, problems of bone deterioration in women are thought to result from changes in their hormone balance after menopause.

The general practitioner sees a very different range of *accidents and injuries* to those which present in hospitals. The family doctor is largely concerned with lacerations and open wounds, and sprains and strains, which are more common among men than women aged 45–64, although women aged 65 and above have greater risks of these than men of the same age; and with bruises and contusions which are more frequent among women in each age group. Side effects of drugs are also more common among women in each age group, reflecting the fact that women are the greater users of GP and pharmacy services.

Perhaps the most interesting disparity between the sexes is in rates of *mental disorder*, but, as we have already seen, the definition of mental illness varied so much between GPs that it is difficult to place

TABLE 7.10   *Rates of mental disorders per 1000 at risk in age groups 45 and above, by sex: England and Wales 1981–2*

Category of condition	Male			Female		
	45–64	65–74	75	45–64	65–74	75+
Serious	7.1	7.9	28.9	10.4	15.1	48.1
Intermediate	34.2	26.8	31.2	69.5	60.7	51.4
Trivial	56.4	51.9	50.0	122.3	111.7	90.7

SOURCE: RCGP, 1986

any weight on the figures. However, as in the previous chapter, we can look at the classification of mental disorder by degree of seriousness of the illness, on the assumption that a serious disorder may be easier to diagnose accurately (Table 7.10).

The GPs clearly identify more serious mental disorders among their patients as the age of those patients rises, which again is not unexpected. Although the *rate* of trivial mental disorders peaks in the age group 45–64, and declines thereafter, such disorders constitute, at around 60 per cent, a constant proportion of all mental illness diagnosed by GPs. Women's rates of mental disorders are twice those of men at ages 45–74 and exceed male rates by over 70 per cent at ages 75 and over.

The bulk of the conditions diagnosed by GPs under the category of *mental disorders* are anxiety disorders, neurotic depressions, insomnia and transit situational disturbances, acute stress reaction, adjustment reaction and, in old age, senility. Women are reported as suffering twice as frequently from all these conditions.

It may be that some doctors are likelier than others to put down women's unexplained symptoms as mental disorders. Figure 6.1 in the previous chapter presented the discharge rates by age and sex from hospitals of those with *signs, symptoms and ill-defined conditions*. Except in the age group 15–44, males predominated. In the GP survey, on the other hand, the rates for conditions under this heading are generally slightly higher for women. It is difficult to avoid the suspicion that men may be referred to a hospital if they have a puzzling symptom, while women may be described as neurotic.

The report of the GP survey also pointed out that those doctors who diagnosed high rates of mental problems among their patients tended to have low rates of *signs, symptoms and ill-defined conditions* – and vice versa. In that category, women aged 45–74 have twice the rate of GP episode for general malaise or tiredness, and much higher rates than men for giddiness, stomach pains and headaches. It does seem that women are genuinely more likely to consult a doctor for these minor conditions, many of which may well be stress-related. The fact that women aged 45–64 have the highest rates of consultation for mental disorders, and also – compared with men – rather high rates for signs, symptoms and ill-defined conditions suggests that many symptoms may be connected with menopause.

But while all this means that we should be careful about accepting claims that women suffer more often from mental illness than men, it does not alter the fact that these women are visiting a doctor for *something*. Their complaints do reflect discomfort of some sort, which contributes to their excess of GP consultations in these age groups.

ILLNESS IN THE COMMUNITY

Consultation with a health professional

The Australian health survey of 1983 (ABS, 1986) suggests that there is much less difference between men and women where consultation with health professionals other than a doctor is concerned. Among those aged 45–64 who had used another health professional in the two weeks prior to interview, there was no difference in the proportion – around a quarter – of men and women who consulted a chemist, or a district, home or community nurse. Men, however, were significantly more likely to have required the services of a physiotherapist (23 per cent compared with 18). Among those aged 65 and over, men were still more likely to have been to a physiotherapist (24 per cent compared with 19 per cent of women) but 29 per cent of the women, and only 26 per cent of men, consulted a nurse.

Medication

Women were, though, significantly more likely to be taking various medications, especially pain relievers and medication for high blood pressure. They were also more likely to have tranquillisers, sedatives or other medication for nervous conditions, and a greater proportion of women than men aged 65 and above were using sleeping pills (Table 7.11).

TABLE 7.11 *Respondents aged 45 and above taking one or more types of medication in two weeks prior to interview, percentages taking each major type, by sex: Australia 1983*

Type(s) of medication	Male		Female	
	45–64	65+	45–64	65+
Common pain relievers	45	36	57	48
Laxatives and stomach medicines	14	21	14	20
Tranquillisers, sedatives, etc.	8	10	11	14
Sleeping pills and medicines	8	16	9	20
Heart, blood pressure, fluid tablets	28	49	39	59

SOURCE: ABS, 1986

Reported ill-health

Women were also more likely than men to report having more than one illness. Among those aged 45–64 who claimed to have experienced some illness in the fortnight prior to the survey, 53 per cent of men, but only 44 per cent of women, said they had suffered from only one condition. Comparable percentages for those aged 65 and over were 38 for men and 32 for women.

SUMMARY AND CONCLUSION

Overall, it does appear that whereas women in the older age groups are less vulnerable to death or serious illness, they have a higher level of minor illnesses, whether measured by GP consultation or by other means. The greatest differentials between these levels of minor illness between men and women appear to be concentrated, above all, in the age group 45 to 64.

The detailed analysis in this chapter does not produce much support for the idea that it is women's greater awareness of potential health problems which leads them to take preventive actions earlier than men, and thus avoid serious illness or death. While it is true that women aged 45–64 have higher rates of GP consultation for all major groups of conditions, and thus may be presenting earlier with some potentially life-threatening disorders, the categories for which they have the largest excess of consultation do not, by and large, involve diseases which lead to death. For instance, they seek treatment for their sinusitis, tonsillitis and so on; it is the chronic bronchitis and emphysema with which men present that are the potential killers.

Some of the excess in the use of doctors and medication among women in this age-group results, once again, from women's different physiology. Problems associated with the menopause; cystitis; and musculoskeletal problems, in particular, are obvious examples. Other conditions for which they seek help have, at least in part, a biological or genetic basis. These include multiple sclerosis and migraine. Many of these conditions are painful, and do much to explain the excess use by women of pain-killing medicines.

Women's different physiology and genetic make-up also account for much of the use they make of hospitals. It is not merely that they have lower hospitalisation rates than men; many of the hospital episodes they do have are for different reasons. In their later forties they are still suffering from pelvic inflammatory disease and other conditions related to their reproductive physiology, including menopause. In their fifties and sixties cancer of the breast and uterus are a major problem. In old age, musculoskeletal problems affect them disproportionately, and lead to many of the falls for which they are also hospitalised.

But the higher levels of women's rates of mental disorder, which appear in hospitals and in the general practitioner reports, remain a puzzle. Linked to it are the questions of why they also have higher reported rates of symptoms which are never diagnosed in general practice, and why they report more health disorders in surveys.

Do older women simply fuss more about their health than older men? It seems unlikely, for two reasons. One is that, as we have seen, there is not much evidence that younger women fuss more than younger men – most of their excess 'illness' results from their particular reproductive problems and different physiology. It is therefore not entirely convincing to assume that they suddenly develop hypochondria after the age of forty-five.

Secondly, the Australian Health survey indicates that there is no difference between the sexes in the percentage who take action if they have identified a health problem: virtually all men, as well as women, who had experienced illness in the two weeks before the survey took *some* action. Thus men do not appear to be more stoical than women.

If there really is more minor illness among women aged 45–64 than among men, what are the possible causes? One possibility may be that much of this illness is stress-related. Men, it has been argued, have a greater range of options in dealing with stress: aggression, use of alcohol, smoking and so on are all more acceptable among males than females. Women, lacking those options, may bottle up their stresses which then appear in the form of headaches, sleeplessness and so on.

Another approach suggests that women in this age group experience more stresses, or different kinds of stress, to those endured by men of the same age. Discussions of stress are complicated by questions of definition and subjective judgement: what to one person might be an intolerably stress-filled existence is, to another, merely pleasantly stimulating. None the less, it is broadly true to say that most of the discussions of stress affecting health have concentrated on aspects – particularly work-related aspects – which, until recently, were more likely to affect men than women. The stresses in women's lives have remained relatively unexplored.

If stress really is an important reason for women's high rates of
mental disorder and unexplained symptoms of illness, then that stress
is not merely confined to older women. While it is true that women
aged 45–64 have the highest rates of reported intermediate or trivial
mental disorder, those rates are only a little above the ones reported
for women aged 25–44. A comparison of Tables 6.9 and 7.10 makes
that point apparent. In other words, we should really consider the
very high rates of reported mental disorder among women in the
whole age span from the mid twenties to the mid sixties.

It would be nice if we could break down the figures a little more, to
see whether there is, for example, a marked difference between
women aged 25–34, and those aged 35–44. This might have helped us
in finding clues to the causes of the problems. As it is, however, there
is no alternative but to talk of the entire age groups 25–64.

There are some contributions to stress in this segment of the
life-cycle which are probably particularly relevant to women. Many
stem from basic demography. These are the years during which a
woman has her children, and has to cope with the responsibilities and
strains which a family involves. Interrupted nights; the quite heavy
physical burden of lifting and carrying; lack of adult companionship
for much of the time: these are only a few of the potential sources of
stress as well as of minor episodes of ill-health.

In her forties she sees the children grow into adolescence and early
adulthood; a period when they are often at their most difficult for a
parent to cope with. The burden, traditionally, falls more upon the
mother. She is also facing a specifically female stress in these years
which has, again, a physiological basis: the menopause, with its
attendant hormonal changes, can create a range of physical and
emotional symptoms. For many women too, it may appear to signal
the end of an important – perhaps the most significant – phase of
their lives.

Among those women in England and Wales aged 50 in 1987,
almost one in five had been divorced (Haskey, 1988). As the
likelihood of divorce has increased, a larger proportion of women has
had to cope alone – at least for some years – with the full burden of
childrearing. Just over half of wives involved in a divorce are under
the age of 35. The number of households headed by a lone parent
with dependent children doubled between 1961 and 1985.

Often, at the same time, the woman is the sole family breadwinner,
and the family's income is likely to be low. In Britain in 1985, almost
two-thirds of lone parent families headed by women were in rented

housing. By comparison, just under a half of lone parent families headed by a man, and only a quarter of married-couple families, had rented accommodation (Haskey, 1987).

Simultaneously, the parents of those aged 45–64 are themselves reaching old age, increasing frailty, and death; here too the problems of providing support fall traditionally more upon daughters (and daughters-in-law) than upon sons. Finally, because of the greater levels of serious illness and even death among men aged 45 and above, a substantial minority of women in the age group 45–64 have to cope with the illness or permanent incapacity of a spouse, or to adjust to widowhood.

This last consideration applies, with still greater force, to women aged 65 and above. Because women tend to marry men older than themselves, and because men have a lower life expectation and greater burden of severe illness, older women are increasingly likely to have an incapacitated husband, or to become widows.

Divorce, and death, added to the small proportion who never marry, leave the elderly with a choice of moving in with other family members, living in an institution or with other people, or living alone. Figure 7.2 shows that more women than men live with some family member until around the age of 60. After that, the percentage of women living in a family declines both more rapidly and more steeply, until only a fifth of women in their eighties live in a family compared to more than two-fifths of men.

At all ages above 45, there are more women than men living alone. Just over half of women in their early eighties live alone, compared with a quarter of men of the same age. After age 85, about a fifth of women live in institutions, almost double the proportion of men in the equivalent age group (Wall and Penhale, 1989). In other words, elderly men are seen as being the responsibility of other family members, while elderly women are more frequently expected to be able to manage alone, or to go into an old people's home when they can no longer do so.

Some of these considerations provide an explanation of at least a part of the use of medical services by older women. Stresses, ranging from those involved in dealing with adolescent children to those caused by the death of a parent, or the divorce or death of a spouse, are quite likely to lead to insomnia, depression or grief. Changes in hormone levels at menopause often themselves create changes of mood, to compound the physical or emotional difficulties associated with it.

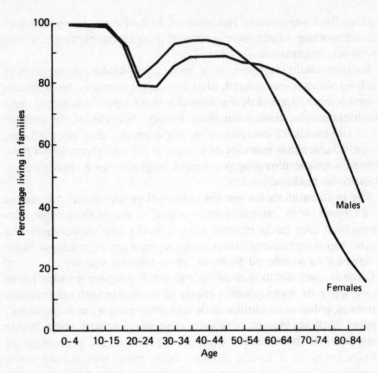

Figure 7.2   Percentage of people living in families, by age and sex: England and Wales 1981.

SOURCE: Wall and Penhale, 1989.

In the longer term, those hormonal changes result in the aches and pains associated with musculoskeletal problems. In an earlier chapter, it was pointed out that much of women's extra life expectation actually meant additional years spent in poor health, often with permanent disabilities. An increasingly restricted life, especially if it involves frequent or constant pain, is not just physically burdensome, but often frustrating and depressing. The depression may be compounded by increasing loneliness, as elderly friends, as well as relatives, die or become incapable of regular contact.

Thus there are grounds for suggesting that older women do indeed suffer stresses which are either not felt by men, or not experienced by them to the same degree. On the whole, it is fair to say that such stresses have not received the same level of attention, or understanding, as stresses which have traditionally affected men: retirement problems, for example.

But, in addition, there may indeed be unrecognised physical illnesses which affect women. Medicine is still primarily an art, rather than a science; a great deal is known about some conditions, a little about many conditions, while still others are only now being 'discovered'. The bundle of complaints for which there is no firm diagnosis, and which, depending on the individual doctor, will be categorised as either inexplicable or a sign of mental disorder, may include genuine sex-specific health disorders.

The problem is that while the symptoms continue to be shrugged off or treated with tranquillisers or antidepressants nobody is likely to know what they really represent. It took a woman to establish that there was a genuine condition of pre-menstrual tension, which involved measurable physical changes such as increase in accident proneness and reduction in ability to concentrate. Osteoporosis may be only one of many conditions which result from post-menopause hormone reductions. Until somebody notices that women, especially women aged 45–64, are complaining about *something*, the statistics represent little more than a big question mark.

8 Reflections on Women's Health

Four hundred years ago in Europe, not even half of a particular birth cohort would survive to maturity. To put it another way, there would be more than 500 deaths before adulthood for every 1000 live births. Only one in every three women lived long enough to take full advantage of her fertile years: two-thirds had died before age fifty. Conditions changed little in most countries until the nineteenth century.

Today, by contrast, in Australia, among every 1000 live births by sex, fewer than 20 males and fewer than 15 females will die before age 18. More than 95 per cent of women born alive will reach age 50; half will survive to age 82. Despite their shorter life expectation, half of all male live births will reach 75.5 years. The pattern in other Western countries is similar.

The reason for the astonishing changes in health and life expectation in the Western world are complex and people still argue about the relative contributions of each. But there is fairly general agreement about the main ones.

Improvements in the water supply and in sewage systems reduced the threat from a number of water-borne or faecal diseases. The hygiene of individuals and families, a well as public hygiene, improved. Housing conditions changed, with fewer people living in damp, dirty and overcrowded hovels or slums. The types of food to which people had access became more varied and often better-balanced.

Transport and communications improved, which meant that although epidemics might spread more easily, reactions to such epidemics could be faster, and containing them became cheaper. In addition, information and education about preventing diseases could be spread more easily, especially with the growth of universal literacy. Working conditions – at least in the past century – have generally improved, and people have shorter working hours and more rest and leisure. People have become more affluent. Spacing of

188

births, and smaller family size, reduced infant, early childhood and maternal deaths.

But perhaps the most important contribution of all came from an increase in education, and especially the education of women. Women were, as one historical demographer explains, 'involved in a much more concrete way than men with all these partial shifts' at the basic level – with making the best of their housing, providing more balanced nourishment to the family, and organising the personal hygiene of family members, for example.

They were the ones who came in closer contact with the bodies of the ill, with infants and children, and they had the final say as to an efficient birth control. It was the dissemination of reading abilities which opened up for the women a new world in all these aspects, which changed their attitudes, increased their knowledge, their motivation. (Imhof, 1986)

Or, as another authority puts it:

once educated, even at a fairly minimal level, girls grew up to be household decision-makers who, through better information, were more efficient in using the limited resources at their disposal to maximise health, particularly the health of their children.

(Mosk and Johanssen, 1986)

In the case of Europe, the transition to low death rates began a century or more ago, so that the evidence about what really happened is rather indirect, and has to be pieced together from often rather inadequate historical sources. But a similar transition has, more recently, been taking place in developing countries; especially since the 1950s, and people have been able to observe the reasons for the declines in death rates more directly.

Here too they have come up with a long list of circumstances which contribute to better health, and here too the one contribution about which everybody seems to agree is women's education. Wherever girls have more chance of access to education (even very basic-level education), lower rates of infant mortality are found.

Exactly how the education of women influences family health is still not clear. Originally, it was assumed that an educated women was simply better-informed about how bodies work and how disease is transmitted and so on, and that she took sensible action on the basis of that better information. However, more recent studies have shown that the effect – declines in mortality – shows up even where the amount of education that girls have received is absolutely minimal. The families of women with just a few years' primary schooling do better, in terms of survival, than those of illiterate women. It does not seem likely that three or four years of education would be enough to provide women with a real understanding of human physiology and disease causation.

More important, probably, are the facts that education changes the woman's attitude to the world, and her status in it.

An illiterate woman remains part of traditional culture, accepting its theories of illness and its attitudes to cure. A young mother with education is allowed to seize a greater share of personal initiative in treating sick children by non-traditional methods . . . She can better manipulate the modern world.

(Caldwell and McDonald, 1981)

One interesting study, based on a rural area of Bangladesh (Lindenbaum, 1983) found that those with primary-school education (often incomplete) and the illiterate mothers continued to share the same traditional beliefs about the causes of illness, and treated sick children in the same ways. A limited amount of education, here, did not seem to have encouraged the mother to explore modern methods of care or cure. What it had done, apparently, was to encourage 'upward social mobility': the women with some education felt that they had achieved a higher social status, and they buttressed their position with a cleaner house, neatness, and better personal hygiene within the family. That in itself was enough to affect the promotion and protection of the family's health.

Whatever the exact mechanisms, the fact remains that all over the world the spread of education to women has a major impact on improving family health and in fostering a decline in mortality rates. As one historical demographer summed up the European past, 'the drastic decrease in infant and child mortality as well as the simultaneous increase in life expectancy . . . above all signifies an enormous *success for women*' (Imhof, 1986).

The curious thing is that women, who have done so much towards improving the overall health of the community, still lose out when it comes to their own health problems.

Issues of women's health, it is probably fair to say, seldom attract much interest among policy-makers or the medical profession. When budgets are being prepared, programmes related specifically to women's health seem, all too often, to be regarded as an optional extra: icing on the cake. Obstetrics has a certain medical cachet – partly because it provides thriving private practices – but most doctors working in women's health or in women's hospitals would agree that they rate rather badly in the medical pecking order.

One argument for the low priority given to women's health issues is that they are less urgent than the problems of men's health. After all, women live longer, don't they? As we have seen, they do: not only in the richer countries of the world but nowadays even in most of the less developed nations. There are admittedly a few South Asian countries with higher female mortality in childhood, in the reproductive years, or even throughout most of the lifespan. Those countries remind us that women elsewhere were not always so lucky; they also remind us of the disproportionate gains women in most of the world have made, as both sexes increase their life expectation. Thus, levels of ill-health among women have largely been seen from the perspective of whether they provide clues to the differences in mortality between the sexes.

And if women have done better than men, and now live longer than men, surely the true priority is to improve men's health? Especially when interventions to deal with male ill-health appear comparatively easy. The causes of much of the excess male mortality are, at least in theory, preventable. Young men die predominantly from accidents or suicide; older men from coronaries. Change male behaviour and many such premature deaths could be avoided.

By contrast, fewer women die premature deaths and those who do are predominantly victims of cancers – above all, breast cancer – whose causes remain largely unknown. The majority of female deaths come at very old ages, and here too the causes of death are more difficult to avoid, or to treat.

That argument has a certain validity, but in concentrating on mortality alone it leaves out far too much of what health is all about. So far as the health of women is concerned, the literature suggests a number of assumptions, some of them contradictory.

The first is that women are or should be generally healthier than men, because of the fact that they live longer. The second is that they nevertheless make a disproportionate use of health services, which indicates – depending upon the viewpoint – either that they take better care of their health than men do, or that they make a lot of fuss about minor conditions. The second assumption, in particular, is based on an underlying framework which is that the health of men and women can be directly compared; that each sex has a similar kind of vulnerability to health impairments.

We have seen that these claims rest on very shaky foundations, bolstered by inadequate, or misleading, statistics. The perspective has often been too 'broad brush' to be particularly informative. Some of the statistics equate use of medical services with ill-health: a proposition which is probably generally true for men, but not for women. Much of the apparent 'excess' use of services by women is for conditions which have nothing to do with ill-health. For example, contraception accounts for a substantial proportion of GP consultations by women, and for the 'medicines' which women say they take.

The use of contraception is only one instance in what is the wider problem of separating preventive health measures from the treatment of health disorders. The statistics in Chapter 5 indicate that it is largely women who go to GPs for general health advice, presumably for their families as well as themselves, as family health care has traditionally been an important female responsibility. Most people – including most health professionals – believe we should be encouraging this kind of contact with the medical profession.

We need, however, to be able to distinguish between consultations for measures like contraception, consultations for preventive health care, and consultations for symptoms of ill-health. Without such distinctions, the picture of the use women make of health services is both inflated and distorted.

This is not just an academic issue. Most women are aware, however vaguely, that they are supposed to be disproportionate users of health services, and many of them visit a doctor with an uneasy feeling that they may be wasting his or her time. Public complaints by doctors about the trivial nature of many of their patients' consultations only reinforce their doubts.

But with increasing emphasis being placed today on preventive medicine and for families to take more responsibility for their own health promotion and protection, the need for health guidance, rather than merely for straightforward diagnosis of symptoms, is likely to grow. As the earlier part of this chapter indicated, it is women who are likely to play the most significant role in family health promotion. If women are to be encouraged to make use of medical services to get guidance in health protection for themselves and their families, it will be important that they do not see themselves

– and are not seen by the professionals – as simply overloading the health services with minor complaints.

Another aspect of the difficulty of separating out preventive health measures is that health practitioners, quite naturally, use their contacts with patients over one issue to carry out health checks for other conditions and provide other health advice.

Take, for example, the person who visits a GP with a sprained ankle. If the GP learns that the damage was done while taking part in some outdoor activity, he or she may take the opportunity to check whether the patient has had a tetanus injection recently. Should the patient explain the sprain as only the latest in a series of recent minor accidents, the GP might suggest an eye test, do a blood-pressure check, or caution against over-weight.

Besides visiting a doctor for a complaint, women in the reproductive years will see the GP for contraception and pregnancy: visits which alert any doctor to considerations of anaemia, blood pressure, weight, smoking, cervical smears, varicose veins . . . Thus women are far more likely than men to be checked and advised by their doctors. A proportion of such women *will* be found to have a condition that needs treatment, and the checks may ensure that any necessary action is taken early enough to prevent more serious health impairment, or even death.

To that extent, the theory that it is women's greater involvement with the health services which gives them greater longevity has some validity. But is it important that, when discussing women's apparently greater ill-health than men's, such doctor-initiated screening should not be used to imply that women disproportionately demand medical services.

Any simplistic assumption, though, that women's greater use of health services protects them from premature deaths from *the same types of illness which men suffer from* does not seem to be borne out by careful examination of the available statistics. The theory depends on the assumption that women notice symptoms and take them at an early stage to a professional who will then cure or control that condition. If that were true we could expect that women would report equal or higher rates of illness from the same diseases that kill men, but this is not the case.

In addition, as we have seen, when the illnesses and causes of death of men and women are grouped under broad diagnostic headings they appear much more similar than in fact they are. To find out whether, and how far, women's health problems are the same as those of men, we have to look in much more detail at statistics which are frequently – and misleadingly – aggregated.

In fact, women have a very different health profile to men, in the illnesses they suffer and those from which they die. There really is a different pattern in female morbidity and mortality, at all ages, which seems to result from a combination of genetic and biological, and behavioural and environmental, factors. In addition, many of their health impairments are linked to their reproductive system, and it is this more complex system which results in much of the reported excess in ill-health.

Fertility and infertility, menstrual and menopausal problems, pelvic inflammatory disease, vaginitis and thrush are the major contributors to women's ill-health in the reproductive and post-reproduction years. First showing up in those years, too, although their most serious manifestations occur later, are breast and cervical cancer – significant causes of female illness and death. In the later years, changes in female hormone levels help to account for women's greater frequency of diseases of the bones and joints. Women have a special vulnerability above and beyond the susceptibility to illness in general which both sexes suffer.

What is a matter for concern is how little this has been reflected in the literature on health differentials. If menstrual problems are reported in the Australian health survey as the seventh most common condition among *women of all ages*, it surely justified being analysed properly so that its importance among those aged 15–45 could be seen.

Studies of the numbers of days men and women take off work, or go to bed, for a health impairment largely rest on an assumption that the risks of ill-health are equal for each sex. That adult women have an *extra* group of conditions, including menstrual and menopausal problems, pregnancies and abortions, is seldom taken into account.

Again, this may be a matter of how health and ill-health are defined. If we see ill-health as something abnormal, something going wrong with the system, then menstruation and pregnancy are not manifestations of ill-health. They are normal biological conditions which happen to women, and, as I have argued, should not be routinely included in data used to measure health impairment.

However, from saying that conditions related to women's fertility are normal, it is very easy to move to the assumption that – unless there is some pathological problem – they do not involve ill-health.

Yet 'normal' pregnancy involves, very often, backache, tiredness, nausea and so on: 'normal' menstruation may involve heavy bleeding, backache, cramps or pre-menstrual tension. Use of contraception may also produce side-effects – headaches, irregular bleeding, and so on.

Women enduring these uncomfortable and even painful symptoms are very far from the WHO definition of healthiness: they do *not* enjoy complete well-being. Discomfort or pain should not be invisible just because they are not symptoms of pathological disease.

We know this in theory: after all, ageing is a 'normal' process which affects most people eventually, but when it manifests itself, for instance, in stiff joints, an erratic memory, or difficulty in reading or hearing, we recognise that these manifestations are health problems for which we would like some intervention. Why, in practice, should it be so difficult to recognise that women from menarche to menopause have special health problems?

It is both obvious and boring to trot out – yet again – the answer that health, like many other things, has been defined largely by men and in male terms, and that the same is true of health care services. However, something which is obvious and boring may nevertheless be true, or at least largely true. The types of research undertaken, statistics which are collected, and the way in which they are analysed and presented, are obviously dependent on the basic judgements which are made about what is significant or important. The lack of attention which has been given to the entire range of issues concerning women's health suggests a fundamental ignorance about, or indifference to, a feminine perspective.

But women themselves may be responsible for part of the invisibility of their condition. Early feminists tended to play down or deny differences between the sexes. This was an entirely necessary counter to the male assumption that women neither could nor should have equality because they were weak and inferior beings. It was also broadly correct, in the sense that the overall similarities between men and women are much greater than their differences. It did mean, though, that such differences as there were became difficult to discuss. Perhaps few people were less sympathetic to complaints of menstrual period pains, for instance, than were some of the first generations of women doctors.

A more recent generation of feminists, anxious to reclaim a certain uniqueness for women, has celebrated the reproductive capacity and some of its implications. Women are the creators of life, the mothers.

Women are the nurturers, of the species as well as the individual. In stressing women's life-giving and often life-preserving roles, they have not been any more anxious than their predecessors to draw attention to the discomforts, stresses and health risks which often go with them.

If the physical problems which result from women's different physiology have often been ignored or played down, so too, I would suggest, have some of the stresses which women face more routinely than men. In Chapter 7 it was argued that these stresses include, for example, some which result from elementary demography, as well as others which are based on circumstances, or on biological vulnerability.

Women in their forties and fifties are faced very often with the need to cope simultaneously with adolescent children and the increasing needs of their own, and their partner's ageing parents, while at the same time some of them have partners who develop incapacity; others will lose their partner altogether: a few through death, and many more because of separation or divorce. Older women often suffer increasing pain from osteoporosis and conditions of the joints; they are very likely to be bereft of a partner, and to live alone as well as, too frequently, in some poverty.

Much of the literature on differential health has focused on male stress (as contributing, for example, to coronory thrombosis and illness or early male death) or has examined stress for both sexes only in terms of people's roles as breadwinners or wage-earners versus, or in addition to, their household responsibilities. There is often the assumption that caring for children involves the same level of stress regardless of the number of children in a family, or their ages, or the amount of support available. Here again it is tempting, but probably too simplistic, entirely to blame the male-world view for such a narrow interpretation of the stresses which may affect women.

Feminists were, for a long time, anxious to demonstrate that women could hold down a job without detriment to their family life: so far as health status is concerned, the statistics suggest that they were quite right. Their more recent concern has been to reassert the importance of woman's childbearing and rearing activities. In doing so, they have identified certain types of stress which women may face, primarily from lack of recognition by society of the significance of their role. Hence the calls for pay for home-work, and that women's currently unwaged activities should be included in measures of national product, for example. But they seem to have been reluctant to go further and look at whether some aspects of caring for a family are intrinsic causes of unwelcome stress. Politically, it may be as difficult for them to admit the possibility that the demands put upon a caring women may be almost intolerable, as it is for the unregenerate upholder of Traditional Family Values.

The experts – demographers, epidemiologists and so on – have also been pretty backward in examining the real issues of women's health in the Western world. As we have seen, the hazards of childhood infections and neglect, and of childbearing, which are still unhappily evident in many third world countries, have virtually been eliminated for women in the industrialised world. Partly as a result, their life expectation has increased dramatically. The contrast between their lives and deaths, and those of women in the poorer countries, shows that much of the illness, and most of the deaths, which third world women suffer are *preventable*. Obviously, finding ways to ensure that they are prevented has had a higher priority with many health professionals than looking in detail at the remaining health impairments elsewhere.

Yet women make up more than half the population. Among those aged 75–84, they form nearly two thirds of the population. On the basis of numbers alone, they deserve more serious attention than they are currently getting. This book has suggested, I believe, that women's health is both better and worse than is usually thought, and that it is in many ways fundamentally different to that of men. That too little is known about women's health problems and needs is apparent not only from existing research but from the rather large proportion of complaints – especially among women in their fifties and sixties – which are inadequately diagnosed. Those complaints mean that women are suffering from something, and are suffering in quite substantial numbers. There is a pool of ill-health among women which is currently unnoticed, let alone explored and mapped.

We need a fuller understanding and recognition of women's health problems, based on increased knowledge, if it is to be possible for all those concerned with women's health to ensure suitable health care, and to enable women themselves not only to have, but also to *enjoy*, their long lives.

References

Adler, M. W. (1982) 'Sexually Transmitted Diseases', in Miller and Farmer (1986).

Alauddin, Mohammad (1986) 'Maternal Mortality in Rural Bangladesh: The Tangail District', *Studies in Family Planning*, vol. 17, no. 1, pp. 13–21.

Armitage, R. J. (1987), 'English Regional Fertility and Mortality Patterns' *Population Trends* no. 47, Spring 1987, pp. 16–23. HMSO, London.

Arriaga, E. E. (1981) 'The Deceleration of the Decline in Mortality in LDCs: The Case of Latin America', in IUSSP International Population Conference, Manila, Ordina Press, Liege.

Australian Bureau of Statistics [ABS] (1979), Australian Health Survey 1977–78, ABS, Canberra, Catalogue no. 4311.0.

Australian Bureau of Statistics [ABS] (1986a) Australian Health Survey 1983; Illness Conditions Experienced, ABS, Canberra, Catalogue no. 4356.0.

Australian Bureau of Statistics [ABS] (1986), Australian Health Survey 1983, ABS, Canberra, Catalogue no 4311.0.

Australian Government Actuary (1985), Australian Life Tables 1980–82, Australian Government Publishing Service, Canberra.

Baghurst, Katrine I. (1986) 'The Relative Health Status of Men and Women – Morbidity or Mortality?', in Kirby-Easton and Davies (1986).

Beacham, Roland (1984) 'Economic Activity: Britain's Workforce 1971–81', *Population Trends*, vol. 37, pp. 6–14, HMSO, London.

Berry, R. J. (1982) 'The Leukaemias', in Miller and Farmer (1982).

Birch, Francis (1979) 'Leisure Patterns 1973 and 1977', *Population Trends*, no. 17, pp. 1–8, HMSO, London.

Bone, Margaret (1986) 'Trends in Pre-marital Sexual Behaviour in Scotland', *Population Trends*, no. 43, pp. 7–14, HMSO, London.

Bourgeois-Pichat, Jean (1978) 'Future Outlook for Mortality Around the World', *Population Bulletin of the United Nations*, no. 11, pp. 12–41, United Nations, New York.

Breeze, Elisabeth (1985) *Women and Drinking*, Office of Population Censuses and Surveys/Department of Health and Social Security, HMSO, London.

Bulusu, Lak and Alderton, Michael (1984) 'Suicides 1950–82', *Population Trends* no. 35, pp. 11–17, HMSO, London

Caldwell, J. C. and Ruzicka, L. T. (1985) 'Determinants of Mortality Change in South Asia', in Srinavasan and Mukherji (1985).

Caldwell, John C. and MacDonald, Peter (1981) 'Influence of Maternal Education on Infant and Child Mortality: Levels and Causes', International Population Conference, Manila, 1981, vol. 2, pp. 79–96, International Union for the Scientific Study of Population, Liège.

Chamberlain, J. (1982a) 'Carcinoma of the Female Breast', in Miller and Farmer (1982).

Chamberlain, J. (1982b) 'Gynaecological Cancers', in Miller and Farmer (1982).

Chamberlain, J. (1984) 'Failures of the Cervical Cytology Screening Programmes', *British Medical Journal*, no. 289, 6 October, pp. 883–4.

Chilvers, Claire (1978) 'Regional Mortality 1969–73', *Population Trends*, no. 11, pp. 16–20, HMSO, London.

Colvez, A., Robine, J. M., et. al. (1986) 'L'espérance de la vie sans incapacité en France en 1982', *Population*, vol. 41, no. 6, pp. 1025–1042, INED, Paris.

Comfort, A. (1979) *The Biology of Senescence*, (3rd edition), Churchill Livingstone, Edinburgh.

Compton, P. A. (1985) 'Rising Mortality in Hungary', *Population Studies*, vol. 39, no. 1, p. 71–86.

D'Souza, Stan and Chen, Lincoln C. (1980) 'Sex Differentials in Mortality in Rural Bangladesh', *Population and Development Review*, vol. 6, no. 2, pp. 257–71.

Daykin, Chris (1986) 'Projecting the Population of the United Kingdom', *Population Trends*, no. 44, pp. 28–33, HMSO, London.

de Scrilli, A. K, et. al. (1986) 'Cigarette Smoking in Pregnancy: Relationship to Perinatal Outcomes in Six Italian Centres', *Genus*, vol. 72, nos 1–2, pp. 37–69.

Department of Health and Social Security and Office of Population Censuses and Surveys [DHSS] (1986) Hospital In-patient Enquiry: summary tables England 1984, Government Statistical Service, HMSO, London.

Dunnell, Karen (1979) *Family Formation 1976*, Office of Population Censuses and Surveys, HMSO, London.

Durkheim, E. (1952) *Suicide: A Study in Sociology*, Free Press, New York.

Dutton, John Jr (1979) 'Changes in Soviet Mortality Patterns, 1959–77', *Population and Development Review*, vol. 5, no. 2, pp. 267–92.

Farmer, R. D. T., Nixon, A. and Connolly, J. (1982) 'Accidents', in Miller and Farmer (1982).

Farrell, Christine (1978) *My Mother Said*, Routledge & Kegan Paul, London.

Finch, B. E. and Green, Hugh (1963) *Contraception Through the Ages*, Peter Owen, London.

Findlay-Jones, Lyn (1986) 'Hysterectomy in Australia: A Social Perspective' in Kerby-Eaton and Davies (1986).

Florey, C. du V. (1982) 'Diabetes Mellitus', in Miller and Farmer (1986).

Fox, John (1982) 'Socio-Economic Differences in Mortality', *Population Trends*, no. 27, pp. 8–13, HMSO, London.

Gardner, Martin and Donnan, Stuart (1977) 'Life Expectancy: Variation Among Regional Health Authorities', *Population Trends*, no. 10, pp. 10–12, HMSO, London

General Household Survey, 1984 (1986), Social Survey Division, OPCS, HMSO, London.

Gove, W. R. and Hughes, M. (1979) 'Possible Causes of the Apparent Sex Differential in Physical Health: An American Observation, *American Sociological Review*, no. 44, pp. 126–146.

200   *References*

Graunt, John (1975) *Natural and Political Observations Mentioned in a Following Index and made upon the Bills of Mortality*, John Martin, 1662; reprint edition Arno Press, New York.

Gwatkin, D. R. (1980) 'Indicators of Change in Developing Countries' Mortality: The End of an Era? *Population and Development Review*, vol. 6 no. 4, pp. 615–44.

Hakulinen, T., Hansluwka, H., Lopez, A. L. and Nakada, T. (1986) 'Estimation of Global Mortality Patterns by Cause of Death', in Hansluwka et. al. (1986)

Hamilton, J. B. (1948) 'The Role of Testicular Secretion as indicated by the effects of castration in man and by studies of pathological conditions and the short lifespan associated with maleness', *Recent Progress in Hormone Research*, no. 3, pp. 257–324.

Hansard (18 April 1985) Written Answers, vol. 77, no. 99, col. 229, HMSO, London.

Hansluwka, Harald, Lopez, Alan D., Porapakkham, Yarawat and Prasartkul, Pramote (1986) *New Developments in the Analysis of Morbidity and Mortality*, World Health Organisation and Mahidol University, Bangkok.

Haskey, John (1987) 'One Person Households in Great Britain: Living Alone in the Middle Years of Life' *Population Trends*, no. 50, pp. 23–31, HMSO, London.

Haskey, John (1988) 'Trends in Marriage and Divorce, and Cohort Analyses of the Proportions of Marriages Ending in Divorce', *Population Trends*, no. 54, pp. 21–8.

Haskey, John and Coleman, David (1986) 'Cohabitation before Marriage; a comparison of information from marriage registration and the General Household Survey', *Population Trends*, no. 43, pp. 15–17, HMSO, London.

Heligman, Larry (1983) 'Patterns of Sex Differentials in Mortality in Less Developed Countries', in Lopez and Ruzicka (1983).

Hetzel, Basil, S. (1983) 'Life Style Factors in Sex Differentials in Mortality', in: Lopez and Ruzicka (1983).

Hetzel, Basil (1974) *Health and Australian Society*, Penguin, Harmondsworth, England and Ringwood, Australia.

Hibbard, Judith H. and Pope, Clyde R. (1983) 'Gender Roles, Illness Orientation and Use of Medical Services', *Social Science and Medicine*, vol. 17, no. 3, pp. 129–37.

Hicks, Neville (1978) *This Sin and Scandal: Australia's Population Debate 1891–1911*, Australian National University Press, Canberra.

Hunt, Audrey (1978) 'The Elderly: Age Differences in the Quality of Life', *Population Trends*, no. 11, pp. 10–15.

Illich, Ivan (1977) *Limits to Medicine – Medical Nemesis: The Exploration of Health*, Pelican Books, Penguin, Harmondsworth.

Imhof, Arthur E. (1986) 'Life-course Patterns of Women and Their Husbands: 16th and 20th Century', in Sorensen, Aage, B., Weinert, Franz E and Sherrod, Lonnie R., *Human Development and the Life Course: Multidisciplinary Prospects*, Laurence Erlbaum, New Jersey and London.

Imhof, Arthur E. (1986a) 'What has Longevity in Europe and Japan to Teach India?', *Demography India*, vol. 15, no. 1, pp. 1–25.

Jeanneret, Olivier (1983) 'Sex Differentials in Mortality and Health Care Delivery: a tentative exploration of some relationships', in: Lopez and Ruzicka (1983).

Johnston, Denis F. (1985) 'The Development of Social Statistics and Indicators on the Status of Women' *Social Indicators Research*, no.16, pp. 233–61.

Khan, Atiqur Rahman, Jahan, Farida Akhter, and Begum, S. Firoza (1986) 'Maternal Mortality in Rural Bangladesh: the Jamalpur District', *Studies in Family Planning*, vol. 17, no. 1, pp. 7–12.

Kane, Penny (1984) 'An Assessment of China's Health Care', *Australian Journal of Chinese Affairs*, no. 11, pp. 1–24.

Kane, Penny (1988) *Famine in China 1959–61: Demographic and Social Implications*', Macmillan, London.

Kazantzis, G. 91982) 'Neoplasms of the Repsiratory System', in Miller and Farmer (1982).

Kirby-Easton, E. and Davies, J. (1986) *Women's Health in a Changing Society*, vols 1 and 2, University of Adelaide.

Kovacs, Gabor T. and Waldron, Kenneth W. (1986) *Sex Preselection: A Review*, Australian Federation of Family Planning Associations (monograph).

Lindenbaum, S. (1983) 'The Influence of Maternal Education on Infant and Child Mortality in Bangladesh', International Centre for Diarrhoeal Disease Research, Dhaka, Bangladesh (mimeo).

Liu Zheng (1986) *Trends and Patterns of Mortality in China*, ESCAP, United Nations, Bangkok.

Lopez, Alan D. (1984) 'Demographic change in Europe and its health and social implications', in Lopez and Cliquot (1984).

Lopez, Alan D. (1983) 'The Sex Mortality Differential in Developed Countries', in: Lopez and Ruzicka (1983).

Lopez, Alan D. (1984a) 'Sex Differentials in Mortality' WHO Chronicle, vol.38, no.5, pp.217–24, World Health Organisation, Geneva.

Lopez, Alan D. and Cliquot, Robert L. (1984) *Demographic Trends in the European Region: Health and Social Implications* World Health Organisation Regional Publications, European Series no. 17, Copenhagen.

Lopez, Alan D. and Ruzicka, Lado T. (1983). *Sex Differentials in Mortality: Trends, Determinants and Consequences*, Australian National University, Canberra.

Lynge, E. (1984) 'Trends and Perspectives in Mortality', in Lopez and Cliquot (1984).

MacFarlane, Alison (1979) 'Child Deaths from Accident: Place of Accident', *Population Trends*, no. 15, pp. 10–15. HMSO, London.

MacFarlane, Alison and Fox, John (1978) 'Child Deaths from Accidents and Violence', *Population Trends*, no. 12, pp. 22–27, HMSO, London.

Madigan, F. C. (1957) 'Are Sex Mortality Differentials Biologically Caused?', *Milbank Memorial Fund Quarterly*, no. 35, pp. 202–23.

Marcus, Alfred C., Seeman, Theresa E. and Telesky, Carol W. (1983) 'Sex Differences in Reports of Illness and Disability: A Further Test of the fixed Role Hypothesis', *Social Science and Medicine*, vol. 17, no. 15, pp 993–1002.

Marsh, Alan (1984) Smoking: Habit or Choice? *Population Trends*, vol. 37, pp 14–20 HMSO, London

McDowall, Michael (1986) 'The Mortality of Agricultural Workers: Using the Thirteenth Decennial Occupational Mortality Study', *Population Trends*, no. 45, pp. 14–17, HMSO, London.

McKee, Lauris (1984) 'Sex Differentials in Survivorship and the Customary Treatment of Infants and Children' *Medical Anthropoiogy*, vol. 8, no. 2, pp. 91–108.

Miller, D. L. and Farmer, R. D. T. (1982) *Epidemiology of Diseases*, Blackwell, Oxford.

Mosk, C. and Johansson, S. R. (1986) 'Income and Mortality: Evidence from Modern Japan', *Population and Development Review*, vol. 12, no. 3, pp. 415–40.

Nathanson, Constance A. (1983) 'Sex Differences in Mortality', *Annual Review of Sociology*, vol. 10.

Nystrom, S. (1980) 'The Use of Somatic Hospital Care Among the Divorced', *Scandinavian Journal of Social Medicine Supplement*, vol. 17, pp. 1–48.

OPCS (1985) 'A Review of 1984' *Population Trends*, no. 42, pp. 1–14. HMSO, London.

OPCS (1985a) *General Household Survey for 1983*, HMSO, London.

OPCS (1986) *Mortality Statistics: perinatal and infant; social and biological factors, England and Wales 1983*, Series DH, no. 15, HMSO, London.

OPCS (1986a) *Mortality Statistics: childhood, England and Wales 1984, Series DH3, no. 19*, HMSO, London.

OPCS (1986B) *Mortality Statistics: accidents and violence. England and Wales 1984*, Series DH4, no. 10, HMSO, London.

OPCS (1986c) 'A Review of 1985' *Population Trends*, no. 46, pp. 1–12, HMSO, London.

OPCS (1986d) *Mortality Statistics, England and Wales 1984*, Series DH1, no. 16, HMSO, London.

OPCS (1986e) *Occupational Mortality 1979–80, 1982–83*, Series DS, no. 6, HMSO, London.

OPCS (1987) 'Adolescent Drinking' *Population Trends*, no. 47, p. 1, HMSO, London.

Peckham, C., Ross, E. M. and Farmer, R. D. T. (1982) 'Congenital Malformations' in Miller and Farmer (1982).

Peckham C., Ross, E. M. and Farmer, R. D. T. (1982a) 'Pregnancy, Childbirth and Perinatal Mortality' in Miller and Farmer (1982)

Petersen, W. (1972) *Population* (2nd edition), Macmillan, New York.

Pollard, John H. (1986) 'Cause of Death in Australia 1971–81', *Journal of the Australian Population Association*, vol. 3, no. 1, pp. 1–17.

Porapakkham, Yarawat (1983) 'Thailand Case Studies on Sex Differences in the Utilization of Health Resources', in Lopez and Ruzicka (1983).

Porapakkham, Yarawat (1986) *Trends and Patterns of Mortality in Thailand*, ESCAP, United Nations, Bangkok.

Pressat, Roland (1981) 'Prospects for the Reduction of Excess Male Mortality in Low Mortality Countries'. paper presented at the ANU/WHO meeting on Sex Differentials in Mortality: Trends, Determinants and Consequences, Australian National University, Canberra 1–7 December.

Ravindran, Sundari (1986) 'Health Implications of Sex Discrimination in Childhood: A Review paper and Annotated Bibliography', World Health Organisation and United Nations Children's Fund, WHO/UNICEF, FHE 86.2, Geneva.

Research in Reproduction (1986) 'Recent Studies in Human Conception', *Research in Reproduction*, vol. 18, no. 2, pp. 1–2. International Planned Parenthood Federation, London.

Rice, Dorothy P. (1983) 'Sex Differences in Mortality and Morbidity: Some Aspects of the Economic Burden' in Lopez and Ruzicka (1983).

Royal College of General Practitioners, Office of Population, Censuses and Surveys, Dept of Health and Social Security, [RCGP] (1986) *1981–1982 Morbidity Statistics from General Practice: Third National Study*, Government Statistical Service, series MB5, no. 1, HMSO, London.

Ruzicka, Ladislav (1968) *Sebevrazednost v Ceskoslovensku z hlediska demografickeho a sociologickeho*, Ceskoslovenska Akademie Ved, Praha.

Ruzicka, Lado T. and Kane, Penny (1985) 'Nutrition and Child Survival in South Asia', in Srinavasan and Mukherji (1985).

Ruzicka, Lado T. and Caldwell, John C. (1977) *The End of Demographic Transition in Australia*, Australian Family Formation Monograph no.5. Department of Demography, Australian National University, Canberra.

Ruzicka, Lado T. and Hansluwka, Harald (1982) 'A Review of Evidence on Mortality Levels, Trends and Differentials Since the 1950s', in WHO, *Mortality in South and East Asia: A review of changing trends and patterns 1950–75*, World Health Organisation, Manila.

Ruzicka, Lado T. and Kane, Penny (1986) 'Nutritional Deficiencies as a Factor in Differential Infant and Child Mortality' in Hansluwka, Harald, et. al. (1986).

Ruzicka, Lado T. and Kane, Penny (1987) 'Trends and Patterns of Mortality in the ESCAP Region: a comparative analysis', *Mortality and Health Issues in Asia and the Pacific*, ESCAP, United Nations, Bangkok.

Ruzicka, L. T. (1986) 'The Elusive Paths of Mortality Transition' in: Hansluwka, Harald, et. al. (1986).

Schofield, Michael (1965) *The Sexual Behaviour of Young People*, Longmans, London.

Shaikh, Kashem, Mostafa, G., Bhuiya, Abbas, Sarder, A. M., Molla, Ibrahim and Wojtyniak , Bogdan (1985) *Vital Events and Migration Tables 1983*, Scientific Report no. 64, Demographic Surveillance system, Matlab, vol. 14, International Centre for Diarrhoeal Disease Research, Bangladesh.

Shelley, E. M. E. R. and Dean, G. (1982) 'Multiple Sclerosis', in Miller and Farmer (1982).

Shettles, L. B. (1964) 'The Great Preponderance of Human Males Conceived', *American Journal of Obstetrics and Gynaecology*, no. 89, pp. 130–33.

Sitwell, Sacheverell (1973) *For Want of the Golden City*, Thames and Hudson, London.

Srinavasan, K. and Mukherji, S. (1985) *Dynamics of Population and Family Welfare 1985*, Himalaya Publishing House, Bombay.

Stern, C. (1973) *Principles of Human Genetics*, (3rd edn) W. H. Freedman, San Francisco.

Stolnitz, George, J. (1956) 'A Century of International Mortality Trends II', *Population Studies*, pp. 23–4.

Tietze, Christopher (1978) 'Sex Ratios of Abortions' *Human Biology*, vol. 20, no. 3, pp. 156–60.

Townsend, Peter and Davidson, Nick (1982) *The Black Report: Inequalities in Health* Penguin Books, Harmondsworth, Middlesex.

Trivers, R. L. (1972) 'Parental Investment and Sexual Selection', in B. Campbell, *Sexual Selection and the Descent of Man, 1871–1971*, Aldine, Chicago.

United Nations Population Division (1983) 'Patterns of Sex Differentials in Mortality in Less Developed Countries', in Lopez and Ruzicka, 1983.

Vance, Rupert B. and Madigan, Francis C. (1956) 'Differential Mortality and the "Style of Life" of Men and Women: A Research Design', in *Trends and Differentials in Mortality*, Milbank Memorial Fund, New York.

Verbrugge, Lois M. (1980) 'Recent Trends in Sex Mortality Differentials in the United States', *Women and Health*, vol. 5, no. 3, pp. 17–37.

Verbrugge, Lois M. (1983) 'The Social Role of the Sexes and Their Relative Health and Mortality', in Lopez and Ruzicka (1983).

Waldron, Ingrid (1982) 'An Analysis of Causes of Sex Differences in Mortality and Morbidity', in Grove, W. R. and Carpenter, G. R., *The Fundamental Connection Between Nature and Nurture* Lexington Books, Lexington, Mass.

Waldron, Ingrid (1983) 'The Role of Genetic and Biological Factors in Sex Differences in Mortality', in Lopez and Ruzicka (1983).

Wall, Richard and Penhale, Bruce (1989) 'Relationships within households in 1981', *Population Trends*, no. 55, pp. 22–6, HMSO, London.

Ware, Helen (1981) *Women, Demography and Development*, Development Studies Centre Demography Teaching Notes, no. 3, Australian National University, Canberra.

Waters, W. E. and Elwood, P. C. (1982) 'Anaemia' in Miller and Farmer (1982)

Whitehead, Margaret (1987) *The Health Divide: Inequalities in Health in the 1980s*, Health Education Council, London.

WHO (1980) 'The Incidence of Low Birth Weight: A Critical Review of Available Information', *World Health Statistics*, vol. 33, no. 3, pp. 197–224, World Health Organisation, Geneva.

WHO, UNICEF (1986) *Health Implications of Sex Discrimination in Childhood*, WHO, UNICEF, Geneva.

Wingard, Deborah L. (1982) 'The Sex Differentials in Mortality Rates: Demographic and Behavioural Factors', *American Journal of Epidemiology*, vol. 115, no. 2, pp. 205–16.

Wood, P. H. N. and Badley, E. (1982) 'Rheumatic Disorders' in Miller and Farmer (1982).

Young, Christabel (1989) 'Life Cycle Experience of Women in the Labour Force', in Pope, David and Alston, Lee, *Australia's Greatest Asset: Human Resources in the Nineteenth and Twentieth Century*.

Young, C. M. and Ruzicka, L. T. (1982) 'Mortality' in *Population of Australia*, vol. 1, ESCAP Country Monograph Series no. 9, United Nations, New York.

Yusuf, Farhat (1985) *Statistics on Patterns of Hospital Utilization by Local and Regional Areas in New South Wales, 1981*, Health Services Information Bulletin no. 7, Department of Health NSW, Sydney.

Index